"The demographic that chan[...]
is now searching for a new approach to aging and Gillian Ranson's
book, *Front-Wave Boomers*, provides rich detail on the lives of older
adults reimagining the elder years. Ranson's research gives a
powerful voice to her generation's fear and inspiration."
       – Moira Welsh, author of *Happily Ever Older:*
          Revolutionary Approaches to Long-Term Care

"In *Front-Wave Boomers*, sociologist Gillian Ranson asks important
questions about individual preparedness for very old age, the
crucial lessons we can learn about aging and ageism from the
devastation of the COVID-19 pandemic, and, finally, what we can
do as individuals, as communities, and as a nation to make aging
a triumph, not a burden. Rooted in the lived experiences of older
Canadians, and integrating current research, *Front-Wave Boomers*
effectively demonstrates what is at stake and why we must act today
to reimagine aging in Canada."
       – Michael Nicin, executive director, National Institute
          on Ageing, Ryerson University

"*Front-Wave Boomers,* and the study from which it draws, is a
tremendous conversation starter about what it means to expect to
be very old – older as a group than any previous generation – at this
time in history in one of the wealthiest and most peaceful countries
in the world."
       – Susan Braedley, associate professor, School of Social
          Work, Carleton University

"Gillian Ranson's intimate portraits of front-wave baby boomers
portray both privilege and precarity in a powerful generation. I
can see myself, my loved ones, my neighbours, and members of my
community so-often overlooked in the stories woven through each
chapter. *Front-Wave Boomers* skilfully explores how to prepare for
very old age, and critically questions how individuals and society
can fundamentally reimagine the future of aging."
       – Jessica Finlay, co–primary investigator, COVID-19
          Coping Study

Gillian Ranson

FRONT-WAVE
BOOMERS

Growing (Very) Old, Staying Connected,
and Reimagining Aging

on
point
PRESS

VANCOUVER | TORONTO

31 30 29 28 27 26 25 24 23 22   5 4 3 2 1

Printed in Canada on FSC-certified ancient-forest-free paper (100% post-consumer recycled) that is processed chlorine- and acid-free.

Library and Archives Canada Cataloguing in Publication

Title: Front-wave boomers : growing (very) old, staying connected, and reimagining aging / Gillian Ranson.

Names: Ranson, Gillian, author.

Description: Includes bibliographical references and index.

Identifiers: Canadiana (print) 20220141673 | Canadiana (ebook) 20220141789 | ISBN 9780774890502 (softcover) | ISBN 9780774890519 (PDF) | ISBN 9780774890526 (EPUB)

Subjects: LCSH: Baby boom generation – Canada. | LCSH: Old age – Social aspects – Canada. | LCSH: Aging – Canada. | LCSH: Ageism – Canada. | LCSH: Older people – Care – Canada.

Classification: LCC HQ1064.C3 .R36 2022 | DDC 305.260971—dc23

UBC Press gratefully acknowledges the financial support for our publishing program of the Government of Canada (through the Canada Book Fund), the Canada Council for the Arts, and the British Columbia Arts Council.

Printed and bound in Canada by Friesens
Set in Zurich and Minion by Artegraphica Design Co. Ltd.
Copy editor: Lesley Erickson
Proofreader: Helen Godolphin
Cover designer: Will Brown
Cover image: Sandis Helvigs

On Point, an imprint of UBC Press
The University of British Columbia
2029 West Mall
Vancouver, BC V6T 1Z2
www.ubcpress.ca

Contents

FRONT-WAVE BOOMERS

Introduction
Setting the Scene

One afternoon in July 2019, Philip and I met at a Calgary coffee shop. We were there to talk about aging, and Philip had a lot to say.

At seventy-one, he was pulling back from his small consulting business, and he was wondering what to do next. It wasn't that he was missing the work (though, during his career, it had "fed his soul"). It was that he now had questions about what might lie ahead.

"So now I'm in this space," he said. "What am I to do? I have energy. I have enthusiasm, but I don't know where it's going ... It's a disquieting time of life, is what it is."

Philip was probably speaking for many people in his age group. At seventy-one, he was at the front wave of the baby boom – the generation classified as those born between 1946 and 1965 that now makes up more than 25 percent of the Canadian population. Those born in 1946 turned sixty-five in 2011. Like Philip, they're now in their mid-seventies. Over the next decades, millions more will be following them as they head much deeper into old age. Philip would not be the only one with questions about how this move would go. "You can be so busy that you don't take any time to figure out where you're going, or where you should be going," he said. "I know that I'm going somewhere else. But I don't know exactly where that is."

Melanie, another front-wave boomer, described herself as "treading water." At seventy-two, with a seventy-six-year-old husband whose health had taken a sudden downturn, she was primarily concerned about housing and sources of support over the long term. She and her husband were living in a house that was too big, in a community that was not particularly sociable and where contact with younger people was hard to establish. "What's going to happen next, and am I going to be prepared to deal with it?" she asked.

In another conversation that summer, Cynthia talked about concerns that were in a different league. At sixty-four, she was younger than Philip and Melanie, but she was in a more precarious position when it came to aging. She was living on a disability pension, on her own, in subsidized housing. She went to aquafit and yoga classes and walked her dog in the dog park. But she had no close social connections.

"I live in poverty, social isolation, with declining health, mental illness," she said. "There's no one who will care for me ... The only thing that gets me out of bed in the morning is my dog." Cynthia said she had "great clarity" about her situation. "I want to speak to you because I want the voice of someone in my circumstances to be heard."

I wanted her voice to be heard, too, along with the voices of Philip and Melanie and as many front-wave baby boomers as I could find. I reached out to them because I was also deeply interested in what they could tell me about aging. I, too, was a front-wave baby boomer, concerned just as much as they were about the future of (very) old age that was to come. Back in 2019, when I spoke with Philip, Melanie, and Cynthia, I was seventy-two, and wondering, as they were, about what might lie ahead. But as a technically retired but still engaged professor of sociology, I had questions that went beyond the personal.

For some time I'd been interested in the massive demographic changes happening in Canada, and what the consequences might be. The latest census, in 2016, revealed that the proportion of people aged sixty-five or older had reached an all-time high, surpassing for the first time the number of children under fourteen. That growth was mostly due to the entry of the baby boomers into the ranks of the old. We were living longer at a time when greatly reduced fertility rates had produced fewer young people than in previous generations. The result was a demographic revolution that researchers, policy-makers, and media pundits were trying to come to terms with.

The baby boomers driving much of the change were not like the generation of elders who preceded them into (very) old age. A whole range of social factors contributed to the differences. We were better educated. Our working lives had been spent in an increasingly information-based economy, so we would be bringing different skills and experiences with us as we aged. More significantly, we had fewer children, if we had them at all, and the geographic mobility shaping our children's working lives often meant that family members did not live close at hand. Mobility also disrupted the stability of neighbourhoods and the proximity of friends. Who would be around to care when this enormous cohort reached the stage of needing care?

As a sociologist, I considered front-wave boomers to be at a critical stage, on the brink of challenging life changes that were likely to have broad social implications. I wanted to find out the extent to which they were prepared, or preparing, for (very) old age. When I got to work in 2019, addressing this question was my primary goal.

BACK THEN, THE MOST popular view of aging, constructed to some extent by front-wave boomers themselves, was that it was a time of freedom and opportunity – at least for the lucky ones. Having retired from paid employment with pensions in hand and in generally good health (and with the expectation that this stage would be long-lasting), they could travel, volunteer, cultivate hobbies, enjoy their families (especially if they had grandchildren), and spend time with friends.

That was the view of aging promoted in the media – along with advice about keeping fit to maintain this lifestyle for as long as possible. Labelled the "third age," this period between retirement and (very) old age was seen as a time when (with careful attention to pursuing a healthy lifestyle) people could enjoy "successful aging." A search for books on "successful aging" on Amazon and other online vendors revealed just how commonplace the idea had become. There was also a whole new category of popular books geared to boomers seeking to reframe – or reinvent – their careers. These new careers were called "encore careers" in a stage that one researcher called "encore adulthood."

Critics of the focus on "successful aging" (and there were many) noted that it might work for the lucky ones, but it excludes those who have health problems and other disabilities, those who struggle financially, those whose families don't fit conventional patterns, those whose lives are difficult in other ways, and those in Indigenous or other communities with quite different perspectives on what successful aging might look like. Those people are aging too. As author and activist Ashton Applewhite put it in a *Globe and Mail* opinion piece, "All aging is 'successful' – not just the sporty version. Otherwise you're dead."

As far as front-wave baby boomers were concerned, that seemed to me to be the crux of the matter. Resolute focus on the period when we might be expected to be healthy and active failed to take account of the fact that, unless death came first, the "young-old" would eventually become very old. Even for the lucky ones, the independence and autonomy we might have prized earlier on would probably diminish. We would enter the "fourth age," and life would change again.

For the front wave of baby boomers in 2019, this fourth age was getting closer. For most, it probably represented everything that "successful aging" was not. Gerontologists Chris Gilleard and Paul Higgs described it as a "black hole." But it was a black hole that, as noted earlier, would soon be absorbing a record proportion of the population, in Canada and elsewhere. Boomers like me, now in our seventies, were the front wave of a cohort spanning twenty years. What would the fourth age be like, for us? Would we be ready for it?

Many things, collectively, could make a difference – including good genes, good health, good finances, and good luck. But from all I had learned, out of past research and the experiences of my own family and friends, I knew that what would make a difference (on top of almost everything else) was our connections to people – connections that were going to look quite different from those of our parents. Unless we died first, the time would come when we were going to need people – to share our lives, give support when necessary, accept (and appreciate) what we were able to give in return, and keep us connected to the wider world. These social ties would be critical. Where we might find them and how they could be sustained as we became very old seemed, to me, to be the big questions.

The background material that helped prepare me was thought-provoking. I learned a lot about baby boomers as a cohort, as a generation who grew up at a particular time in history that would shape our life experiences and our thoughts about the future. Our passage through that period was distinctive; along the way, it produced many changes – in family life, in communities, and in social connections – that would make our old age different from that of our elders. It also became clear to me that we were aging in a society in which views about old age were often patronizing, if not unkind. Baby boomers were experiencing a lot of criticism. Ageism was all around us, and we often internalized it. That, too, would shape our experience of very old age.

ALL THIS WAS INFORMING my thinking as I started research in earnest. I knew that front-wave boomers were not a homogeneous group. Though we had grown up and into old age at the same time, we hadn't all experienced it in the same way. I wanted to talk to people living in different circumstances and regions across the country, people whose backgrounds were as diverse as I could find.

I wanted to know how prepared they were for old age, which was rapidly approaching, and, in particular, the people who would be in their lives to support them. Informed by my reading, I had many questions. I wanted to hear about their family ties, their friendships, and their educational and work backgrounds (a telling link to current and future financial status); I wanted to know how they were spending their time and the state of their health.

Between May and December 2019, with the help of community organizations, seniors' centres, personal and professional networks, and word-of-mouth referrals, I located and spoke with more than one hundred people across the country, ranging in age from sixty-two to seventy-seven (with an average age of sixty-nine). There was a roughly equal number of women and men. About half were currently married or partnered, about 80 percent had children, and about 10 percent were single and without children. There were also differences in terms of educational and work backgrounds, income level, sexual orientation, and ethnic or cultural identity. They all had decades of adult life experience to share. Along with their backstories, I got a clear sense of their present circumstances, particularly the people in their lives. Given my interest in their preparedness for the years to come, we also looked ahead. Our conversations were immensely rewarding. They gave me a rich and detailed base of information to draw on, and after reviewing it in the early months of 2020, I was prepared to write the book.

I didn't anticipate that a global pandemic would force challenging life changes on everyone – and a widespread shift in thinking about aging. Not surprisingly, COVID-19 also forced a shift in my own thinking. How would the pandemic affect the lives of the people I had spoken with and others like them across the country? How would it affect their current experience, as aging baby boomers, and their thinking about what was to come?

THE PANDEMIC WAS DECLARED in March 2020. Public health authorities focused on "seniors" as a homogeneous group whose members were considered equally vulnerable to COVID-19. Quebec premier François Legault's March 14 request to people over seventy not to leave their homes unless necessary was perhaps the most explicit example of a concern that was widely articulated.

The pandemic's most devastating impact in Canada during the first wave was in long-term care homes, which became hotbeds of infection with alarmingly high death rates. (By May 25, 2020, 5,324 long-term care residents had died of COVID-19 – 81 percent of all COVID-related deaths.) The crisis brought attention not only to the quality of care available in such institutions but also to the experiences of the overworked and underpaid workers who were hired to provide it. Care of the very old, in Canada and elsewhere, began to receive the kind of attention that would surely cause front-wave baby boomers (who might be next in line to need care) to take notice.

All of this seemed likely to push those I had spoken with to confront their age in new ways. Financial worries and health concerns were likely to increase the longer social isolation continued. And, most important from my perspective, the social connections available to them would likely shape how they experienced the constraints of lockdown in their communities.

Local responses to the pandemic would likely shine a bright light on strengths and weaknesses, resources and deficits in the homes, families, and neighbourhoods of the people I had spoken with. They might, in some ways, foreshadow what was further down the road. I wondered if the material I had gathered in 2019 might now be telling only part of the story. It seemed important to add a second goal to the research: to find out what lessons about aging might be learned from the pandemic.

One way to find out was to follow up with my participants, and between March 2020 and March 2021, that's what I did. Having committed to keeping them informed about the progress of the research,

I had already arranged to send update messages. But the messages during the pandemic became check-ins as well as updates. Nearly everyone responded, at least once, often two or three times, over the course of 2020 and beyond, to let me know how they were doing. I also contacted a representative group of some thirty participants, who agreed to more frequent check-ins by phone (or Skype or Zoom).

The check-ins were revealing. During the first wave, there was anxiety but also resolve and a willingness to make the best of what everyone hoped would be a health crisis of short duration. Most people thought they would manage.

The summer of 2020, when restrictions lifted, was a welcome reprieve. But as fall and winter approached and we experienced the second and third waves, resolve often led to COVID fatigue.

For those with the resources to access it, technology such as Skype and Zoom enabled connections that, while not ideal, were better than nothing. As one participant put it: "I can't imagine what an extended lockdown would be like if it happened ten years ago. As much as I'm getting tired of Zoom, I have to say I'm very thankful for it."

But while all participants had at least minimal online access (or at least a telephone), social isolation was a real concern for some. By the time of our last conversation, one self-professed introvert was barely leaving his house. Another was committed to getting outside and walking, but apart from some distant family connections, there seemed to be no people with whom he was in close touch.

In the meantime, Canadians were dealing with media reports on the pandemic's consequences, particularly among the very old. The heavy death toll in long-term care homes had alarmed seniors' organizations and advocacy groups, and led to reports calling for wide-ranging structural and institutional change in care provision. But changes instigated in some provinces were not enough to prevent a second spike in cases in long-term care settings, and more deaths. Indigenous communities were also found to be particularly vulnerable.

Another grim consequence of the pandemic in long-term care settings was the social isolation enforced on residents to reduce infection rates. The media reported often on anxious family members unable to visit elderly residents and accompanied their reports with images of residents, shut in and dependent on (intermittent) contact with care workers to sustain them. These images drew public attention to social isolation in a way that had perhaps never happened before.

But it wasn't only in residential settings that alarm bells were ringing. The mental health effects of the pandemic were recognized by health care workers and family members, among others, to be widespread, and social isolation, particularly among older people, was a rising concern. The availability of social resources, always known to be important, now achieved much greater significance.

In this sense, the pandemic was a case study. It was demonstrating all too effectively what happens when our existing *social* resources are put to the test. It exposed major faults in the care system, among other social problems. And, as months passed with endless media coverage of the crisis, a pattern of heightened ageism began to emerge.

Viewing the pandemic as a case study from which lessons could be learned was a useful way for me to frame the information I had gathered in my follow-up work and fulfill the project's second goal. The people who took part in my research could be viewed as participants in the case study. They had valuable insights to offer. With differential access to social supports and relationships, some managed well (often rising to the occasion as helpers and supporters). Some managed, albeit with occasional concerns and anxieties. And some did not do well. There were lessons to be learned from all of them.

IN EARLY MARCH 2021, as vaccination programs were getting underway across the country, I was ready to end the follow-ups and move on. I now knew much more about front-wave baby boomers – as a cohort with a distinctive history and as individuals with diverse resources and needs. It was time to think more deeply about what I had learned and to look ahead, once again, to the future of (very) old age in postpandemic Canada.

Thinking about what we front-wave boomers might want in our own very old age led me to think more about who we were. Who we were would have a lot to do with what we might want and what we would be willing to settle for. I knew we were not a homogeneous group, and I remembered the observation that not everyone who lives through the same period experiences it in the same way. But we had, collectively, lived through times that were different from those experienced by the generation before us, and we'd experienced a social world that had changed with us. There would be some shifts in our experience and our thinking about very old age.

The pandemic gave us a graphic picture of a particular *kind* of very old age – the kind lived in congregate settings, like long-term care facilities. It probably confirmed our conviction that this was not the way we intended to spend our final years. (Indeed, a survey conducted in July 2020 found that almost 100 percent of respondents sixty-five years and older planned to support themselves so they could live safely and independently in their own homes for as long as possible.)

But neither would we want to be lonely and isolated, like some of the older people whose stories came to our attention during the pandemic. We would want agency and autonomy. And if we lived long enough to need care, we would want it delivered by people who could appreciate and value us as individuals worthy of care.

By March 2021, when I was preparing to move on, these concerns were becoming part of an unprecedented society-wide conversation about elder care and aging. If we front-wave boomers had ideas about what we wanted, others did too. Those advocates and researchers who had sounded the alarm bells were getting more public attention; thoughtful analyses about what needed to change were emerging, along with recommendations and models for doing things differently.

These urgent conversations had the potential to change the environment in which the next generation of elders would grow very old. I needed to take this potential for change into account and to ask whether what I had learned about front-wave baby boomers fit with the different future that seemed to be taking shape. Putting these two pieces together, at a time when answers were sorely needed, became the third and final goal of this book.

THESE THREE GOALS DROVE the book's structure. The first four chapters elaborate on my pre-pandemic goal – to paint a picture of front-wave baby boomers, in all their diversity, and explore their readiness for (very) old age. Chapters 5 and 6 take up the book's second goal – to find out what lessons might have been learned about aging – and ageism – during the pandemic as social and other resources were put to the test and differences in people's situations became clear. The final two chapters take up the book's third goal – to look to the future and to examine both the challenges and the changes that might lie ahead in the field of aging and eldercare. In Chapter 7, I explore the possibilities for doing things differently (now an urgent part of research and policy discussions) in the context of the diverse needs and resources of front-wave baby boomers who will be experiencing those changes first-hand. This is a critically important but often overlooked perspective, which I explore in more detail in Chapter 8. Here I also put forward some strategies – at the personal and social level – for reimagining aging.

BY THE TIME OF MY LAST check-in with Philip, Melanie, and Cynthia, well over a year had passed since our first conversations. It was illuminating to see what could happen, even in a year, on our aging journey.

Philip was dealing with an emptying nest and preparing to sell the family home. He was also searching for new ways to direct his energy and enthusiasm. In his last email, he wrote: "I still am missing something to strongly latch on to which expresses my need to help the present environmental and social challenges of our time." But he also noted a recent Zoom call with a group who recognized and echoed his feeling. He reconnected with them often. "So I'm not alone, which helps."

There had been ups and downs in Melanie's life too. Her husband's health had improved, but there had been a death in the immediate family. She was still thinking about next steps in terms of housing, but long-term care homes would not be in the picture. As she put it, "If I ever needed one more reason why I will not be going to one [it's] the effects of COVID."

Cynthia reported doing a bit better after our initial conversation, but in response to one of my invitations for a follow-up, she told me she was depressed and not up to chatting. So I was delighted to get a more positive response to a later check-in and to learn that people had been reaching out to her. She wrote: "I am doing well! Thankfully I am able to join a small yoga class two times a week. I also forced myself to accept an invitation from friends in [city] to join them in their 'bubble.' I have been there for three week-long visits and it has helped immensely. Not feeling so isolated. Other long ago friends have connected too – strange times."

In my case, big life changes came from a happy source. Just weeks before the pandemic was declared, I became a grandmother. That long-awaited grandchild's arrival led, in short order, to major downsizing and an interprovincial move. For the first time in many years, I had family members close at hand, with all the potential for the giving and receiving of support that our geographical separation had long prevented. And I could be a grandmother-on-the-spot – a role I relished. At the same time, I faced the challenge of getting to know a new community and making new friends.

As it turned out, this has been, for me, a time of surprising growth and change. But I know it won't last forever or even, possibly, for long. I, too, am heading into very old age, when things will change again. But as I've discovered, I'll have some great companions on the journey. Their stories are at the heart of this book.

1

Background on the Boomers

Baby boomers will soon be heading into very old age in unprecedented numbers. To understand what this looming future might look like, we need to know much more about them – what might make them distinctive as a cohort growing up and aging in a particular historical period.

The best and obvious place to start is the period when they were born. In the words of historian Doug Owram, it was the right time, for many reasons. He went on to write a book about Canadian baby boomers to illustrate why they were so fortunate – and so influential.

Owram prefaced his book by noting how rare it was, historically, for people to think of themselves in terms of their generational identity, and for children and adolescents to have such a profound influence on the larger society in which they were growing up. But, he argued, that was the case for the baby boomers, for three main reasons.

The first was the sheer size of their generation. Between 1945 and 1946, Canada saw a 15 percent increase in births. This trend lasted for twenty years and saw more than 8 million babies born in Canada. Live births rose from a low of 227,000 in the mid-1930s to more than 353,000 in the mid-1940s, to a peak of 479,000 by the late 1950s. The baby boom transformed the age balance in the Canadian population. First as babies, then at every age as they grew up, baby boomers constituted what Owram, quoting another historian, called "the pig in the python." At every stage of their young lives, their numbers required major social transformation.

The second reason for baby boomers' influence was that they grew up in prosperous times. The immediate postwar period saw almost unprecedented economic growth. The standard model of the 1950s family, with father as breadwinner and mother as homemaker, came about at least partly because of the number of families that could manage on a single breadwinner's earnings. This economic security allowed society, and parents, to focus on children, something that had not been possible in earlier decades of Canadian family life.

Another feature of family life during this period was its relative stability. In 1961, 94 percent of the 7.8 million children in Canada lived with married parents – the highest proportion observed over the past century. And while greater stability of family life would not necessarily guarantee the happiness of all its members, it did mark a significant, and potentially consequential, shift.

The third reason for boomers' influence was that they were linked to a turbulent decade. As Owram puts it: "Much of the myth, and hence the power, of the baby boom lies in its connection with the fabled decade of the 1960s. Hippies and dope, free love, flower power and women's liberation, Vietnam, the Kennedys and [Pierre Elliott] Trudeau, university protest and the Beatles – the decade has few rivals as an age of change and excitement." This was the decade during which the oldest baby boomers came of age, and, in Owram's view, their experiences gave them the sense that they were different, not just in terms of numbers and opportunities but in character as well. They were expected to *make* a difference.

BY 2019, CANADA HAD been transformed by aging baby boomers into a (demographically) older society. To put it more vividly, the baby boomer "pig" was now headed to the end of the python. They were approaching very old age. How that future "fourth age" would go would be significantly shaped by the past they had experienced, both as individuals and as members of a generation growing up during a particular time.

Sociologists who study aging call this a life-course perspective. One key principle is that "large events such as depressions and wars, or the relative turbulence or tranquility of a historical period, shape individual psychology, family interactions and world views." Some of the enduring transformations in Canadian social and cultural life that emerged during the baby-boom years cast long shadows.

Consider family housing. Greater prosperity and larger families influenced the development of suburbs in major Canadian cities. As Owram notes, "hundreds of thousands grew up, as had their parents or grandparents, in city homes, rural farmhouses, or small villages," but the suburb was "the great phenomenon of the age and came to typify the childhood of the baby-boomer."

The house in the suburbs came to represent a cultural ideal of family living that persisted well beyond that initial baby-boom growth. In the early years, it also reconstituted traditional family connections. Apart from the fact that children outnumbered adults in most neighbourhoods, parents and children lived apart from older family members. Isolated nuclear families were the new norm. And they generally lived in neighbourhoods made up, in terms of socio-economic status and race or ethnicity, of people just like them.

The baby boomers also sparked a transformation in education. The years from 1952 to 1965 – the older boomers' school years – saw increased pressure on the public education system. More schools were needed to accommodate unprecedented numbers of children. There was also a growing sense, among postwar parents, of the importance of their children getting a good education.

This reworking of the education system had several effects. For the first time, classrooms were segregated by age. As Owram observes,

"In earlier generations the predominance of the small school meant that the 'child' in the row next to you might be three grades ahead and three or four years older. As schools exploded in size, and as consolidation took hold, that changed. The grade system, finely dividing children by age, reinforced and further refined the identity of one's peer group."

Another effect was the emergence of a pronounced youth culture as baby boomers reached adolescence. When the parents of baby boomers went to school, most children could be expected to finish Grade 8. But high school beyond that level was still for the most privileged. As late as 1951, the majority of fourteen-to-seventeen-year-olds were not enrolled in school. Baby boomers had different expectations. By 1954, more than half of fourteen-to-seventeen-year-olds were in school, and by the early 1960s that percentage had risen to three out of four. High school became an important focus of this new culture and in various ways set up baby-boom teenagers for the dramatic changes of the 1960s.

In high school, they were subjected to a curriculum that introduced them to ideas about democracy and social justice – an important and perhaps not surprising postwar legacy. And it was in their high school years that they became exposed to the other great innovation of the later 1950s – rock and roll. Young people's music emerged as a force and would grow even more powerful in the decade to follow.

WE IDENTIFY THE BABY boomers with the drama and excitement of the 1960s, but they didn't all experience the decade in the same way. The perception is that they were *responsible* for the drama and excitement, but Owram suggests another view, that "however much the baby boom was a force within the decade, so too were events of the decade crucial in shaping the history of the baby boom."

Whereas questioning authority might have seemed dangerous during wartime, and premature during the time of peaceful recovery in the 1950s, it was both possible and called for in the 1960s, a decade defined by challenges to American policy on the Cold War and communism and events such as the Cuban Missile Crisis and the Vietnam War. Challenges to authority also came from the civil rights movement and the women's movement, which had their roots much earlier than the 1960s. In Canada, this was also the era of the Quiet Revolution in Quebec.

So there was a lot in the world, and at home, to be concerned about – and a generation of young people, the beneficiaries of prosperous times and an education that had taught them to value democracy and challenge injustice, was ready to take up the fight.

Not all baby boomers joined the revolution. The action happened, in Canada as elsewhere, mainly on university campuses. And though university attendance was much higher by the early 1970s than it had been in earlier decades as the baby-boom "pig" reached postsecondary age, only one in six eighteen-year-olds had enrolled. But this was a generation raised to value and identify with their peers. Though not all boomers went on marches or joined boycotts, there were other things they shared such as clothes, music, or drugs – all features of the hippie-led counterculture. As Owram writes, "This was, after all, 'the' generation, and the sense of being involved in a vast peer-group revolution was very very powerful."

Changes also happened in the world that boomers did not create or contribute to, but that would greatly influence their future lives. The publication in 1962 of Rachel Carson's enormously influential book *Silent Spring* and the stunning 1968 photograph *Earthrise*, taken from outer space by a US astronaut, marked the start of the present-day environmental movement.

Another change, with implications much closer to home, was the development of the birth control pill. It was first introduced to Canada in 1960, though at the time it was illegal to advertise or sell any form of contraception. Doctors could prescribe it only for therapeutic, not birth control, reasons. But with growing pressure from the medical community and the public at large, the law was changed in 1969. In effect, contraception was decriminalized. That same year, following Pierre Trudeau's famous comment that there was "no place for the state in the bedrooms of the nation," homosexuality was also decriminalized. (Sadly, decriminalization did not end homophobia and discrimination against the LGBTQ2S+ community.)

BY THE EARLY 1970S, the oldest baby boomers had reached their mid- to late twenties. The country in which most of them had grown up had changed, at least partly thanks to them. Owram summarizes it neatly:

> In some cases, as in the women's movement, environmentalism, and gay rights, issues raised in the 1960s gained momentum. In other instances issues ceased to be controversial simply because they had been accepted by society as a whole – premarital sex being one obvious example, and rock music another ... Older Canadians picked up notions that had originally been identified with youth, and youth found that maybe there were those over thirty who could be trusted after all.

The baby boomers moved into jobs and (later than their parents) started families of their own. And all this, too, was happening in a changing world. For one thing, the prosperity of the 1960s was giving way to greater economic uncertainty. Getting – and keeping – a job became more important.

Most of them, however, managed to do just that. A Statistics Canada study of the working lives of baby boomers between 1983 (when the oldest were in their thirties) and 2010 (when they were in their sixties) found that about two-thirds had entered their fifties in jobs they had held for at least twelve years. In fact, most had worked for the same firm or organization for far longer – often twenty years or more – and even this was considered an underestimation, since most had started their longest job before 1983. This suggests working lives that were quite stable. (By contrast, one-quarter of the sample had more mobile working lives and lower annual earnings and years of pensionable service.)

Advances in technology created other workplace changes. Even the oldest of the baby boomers were part of an economy that, over the decades from the 1970s, became increasingly computer-dependent and knowledge-based. Using Canadian census data from 1971 to 1996, researchers found that this trend was widespread across industries and occupations. Exposure to computer technology was, of course, job-dependent to some extent, but the work experience of many front-wave boomers made them comfortable with information and communications technology outside of work as well.

One of the most substantial changes to the Canadian labour market during the working lives of the boomers was the participation, en masse, of women. In the early 1950s, about one-quarter of women aged twenty-five to fifty-four participated in the labour market (which meant that they either had a job or were looking for one.) In contrast, virtually every man in the same age group was participating. From 1953 to 1990, the labour force participation rate for women grew steadily, rising from about 24 percent in 1953 to 76 percent by 1990. Women's growing workforce participation led to a significant increase in their earnings, which more than doubled between the mid-1960s and 2010. More women were working full-time and in well-paid occupations.

Women's greater participation in paid work and the influence of the women's movement signalled a shift in ideas about family roles too. This shift was reflected in two pieces of legislation enacted in the 1960s. The first, as noted, was the introduction of the pill and the decriminalization of contraception in 1969, which paved the way for family planning in a way not available to earlier generations. Fertility rates began a decline – from an average of 3.1 children per woman in 1965 to 1.6 per woman by the mid-1980s. The second was the 1968

Divorce Act, which extended the grounds for divorce to include a no-fault option based on separation of at least three years. The legislation signalled a shift in the way people perceived marriage. Within a decade, the rate of·divorce in Canada increased six-fold. (There was another spike in 1986, when the minimum separation period was reduced to one year.)

More divorces meant more remarriages. By 1997, 34 percent of marriages involved at least one spouse who had been previously married and, in almost half these cases, both spouses had been married at least once before. In many cases, divorced parents brought children to new partnerships. In 1994–95, nearly 9 percent of Canadian children under the age of twelve lived in a stepfamily.

THESE TRENDS AFFECTED baby boomers born and raised in Canada to settler families – the majority, in demographic terms. But they were joined, over the years, by boomers from many other countries. Immediately after the Second World War, the immigration boom mostly favoured people from the United Kingdom. But the 1950s to the 1970s also saw the arrival of immigrants from Germany, the Netherlands, Italy, Greece, Yugoslavia, and Portugal.

World events also led to the massive movement of refugees and migrants from different parts of the world to Canada. Examples included the arrival of 60,000 boat people from Vietnam, Cambodia, and Laos in the late 1970s; 85,000 immigrants from the Caribbean (for example, Jamaica, Haiti, and Trinidad and Tobago) and Bermuda in the 1980s; 225,000 immigrants from Hong Kong over the ten years leading up to its return to China by the United Kingdom in 1997; and 800,000 immigrants from India, the Philippines, and the People's Republic of China in the 2000s. All had experiences that differed from the majority of Canadian baby boomers who grew up in stable, suburban-dwelling, predominantly white households.

The experiences of boomers born to Indigenous parents also differed in sobering ways. In 1966, when white boomer children were sitting in suburban classrooms, twelve-year-old Chanie Wenjack was running away from his residential school near Kenora, Ontario. He died in the attempt, from hunger and exposure. Chanie, an Anishinaabe boy, had grown up on an Ontario reserve and was sent to a residential school with three of his sisters when he was nine. His death sparked national debate and led to the first inquest into the treatment of Indigenous children in residential schools. The (non-Indigenous) jury concluded: "The Indian education system causes tremendous emotional and adjustment problems for these children." They recommended that "a study be made of the present Indian education and philosophy. Is it right?"

It took until 1996 to close the last residential school, after some 150,000 students had passed through the system. It's hard to say how many, like Chanie Wenjack, were of baby boomer age, but it's likely a good proportion of Indigenous people aged sixty-five and older in Canada today share a residential school background.

Some might also have endured other forms of family trauma related to the so-called Sixties Scoop, which saw Indigenous children removed from their families and communities – often without their parents' or bands' consent – to be adopted into predominantly non-Indigenous families across Canada and the United States. Estimates vary, but recent research has found that more than twenty thousand children may have been affected – often with serious psychological and physical consequences.

FROM THIS HISTORY, it was clear to me that front-wave baby boomers would be approaching very old age with highly diverse backgrounds. Life did not unfold uniformly even for those doted-on baby boomers who'd grown up in stable suburban homes and youth-oriented communities.

A life-course perspective also recognizes that people have agency; they make choices within the constraints and opportunities available to them. Educational and job opportunities put people on different paths. So, too, do relationship choices, the presence (or absence) of children, and other social supports. Life paths are also affected by gender and race. And people are linked. The bonds of kinship link generations, and we connect with people at all stages of our lives. Our lives are "embedded in relationships with people, and are influenced by them."

For baby boomers approaching very old age, these relationships would be critical. Important as other dimensions might be – health, financial security, and physical safety being the main ones – it is people who would make a difference. With this in mind, I used the baby boomer background information I gathered to examine relationship issues that might make our experience of very old age different from that of our own elders.

Demographically, as our spiking divorce rate suggests, front-wave boomers were less likely to stay married, if we married at all. In a study of divorce in Canada, sociologist Rachel Margolis and her colleagues found a tendency for couples to divorce later in life and noted that baby boomers have "more tumultuous marriage histories" than previous generations. They are the group most likely to have experienced divorce and most likely to be currently divorced (about 10 percent, in 2018). Later-life divorce is another feature of some boomer families, though the trend is less marked in Canada than in the US.

Though a high proportion of baby boomers had children (around 90 percent by their mid- to late sixties), we had fewer of them. And those children – many of them millennials facing their own challenges – are also having fewer children and at a later age. This has had obvious implications for baby boomers, whose transition to grandparenthood might be delayed – or might not happen. In the mid-2010s, while upwards of three-quarters of people in their late sixties and early seventies were grandparents, some had been grandparents-in-waiting for quite a while. Overall, boomers have far fewer family connections than our forebears did.

Even for those boomers who do have children and grandchildren, contact with other family members might not always be straightforward. The constraints of work in a global economy – and women's greater participation in it – might leave little time for family support. Work commitments might also mean that families are geographically dispersed. Transnational migration might separate families even more dramatically. Family connections can also be shaped by relationship breakdowns and divorce. And in families across the board, relationships might not always be warm and supportive. Finally, there is a significant minority of front-wave boomers who have neither children nor grandchildren, now coming to be known in the research literature as "elder orphans." For them, relationships outside their families might be the most significant.

So where might those relationships be found?

Our parents tended to find connection and support in the communities where they lived. But by the time we were approaching very old age, communities, just like families, were changing. The house in the suburbs had been a draw for boomers raising families, just as it had been for their parents, and many older boomer couples still lived in the suburbs. But in physical, geographical terms, the suburbs might now be less stable, more car-dependent, and less familiar than the sociable, interconnected neighbourhoods – the "communities of place" – they had once been. And not all older boomers have partners. According to census data, in 2016, some 28 percent of households in Canada were single-person. More than a quarter of them housed people over sixty-five. Neighbours didn't always know neighbours.

Of course, communities of place were not the only communities around when I embarked on my research. Social ties had been transformed by the internet, social media, and the mobile connectivity of cellphones. Evidence suggested that older baby boomers were making good use of these information and communications technologies (ICTs for short). Many had experience in workplaces where they were commonplace. As one group of Canadian researchers commented:

"To an appreciable extent, it is not so much that the aged have started using ICTs, but that long-time users of ICTs have grown into older age."

But who they might be connecting *with* raised questions and concerns. Other research suggests that as baby boomers age, they tend to have fewer personal connections close at hand and, significantly, fewer connections to younger generations. That, too, would impact their experience of aging.

AS IT TURNED OUT, the people who agreed to speak with me represented a richly diverse set of life experiences and backgrounds. Where people grew up, the cultural context of the 1960s, the constraints they faced, and the choices they made about school, work, and family – all of these things, among others, did indeed foreshadow what came later for many.

Of all my participants, Sam's was the story that most closely fit the popular image of the turbulent, exciting 1960s. Sam was seventy when we met. Born in San Francisco, he came of age as the hippie movement was emerging. He joked about seeing a T-shirt whose message read: "I may be old, but I saw all the great bands." (The message resonated – he listed seeing the early concerts of Jefferson Airplane, Janis Joplin, and Led Zeppelin.) But he also remembered participating in the protests that were another feature of San Francisco life. He described the scene as "a real eye-opener, culturally and in a whole lot of ways."

Sam was also representative of the group of Americans who fled to Canada to avoid being drafted to fight in the Vietnam War. He was twenty when he arrived, and when his first relationship broke down (and when amnesty had been declared for draft dodgers), he returned to the United States to complete a university degree. He then came back to Canada, started a new family, embarked on graduate studies, and became a college instructor – a job he held till he retired.

Mary, also seventy when we first spoke, grew up in an upper-middle-class family in Toronto and had what she described as a fairly typical 1950s upbringing until her high school years, when she, too, became involved in protest movements. She opposed the Vietnam War, was involved in an antipoverty coalition, then dropped out of university after her second year to live (briefly) in a commune. In 1975, after five years away, she returned to university and, like Sam, embarked on graduate studies, which led to an academic career. When we spoke, she had a partner, two daughters, and three grandchildren. She was a devoted grandmother.

These classic 1960s coming-of-age stories were the exceptions, though. Gary went from high school in southern Ontario to training as an electrician, marriage at twenty, then a long-term job in a steel mill. Janet grew up in Saskatchewan, married at twenty, and did secretarial work while her husband was at university. Later, she balanced caring for her two children with working as an office administrator, selling real estate, and taking courses to train in home design. She later worked with a realtor, staging houses for sale.

Tariq was born in India and immigrated to Canada in 1972, when he was twenty-three. He had completed a bachelor of commerce degree in India, but his first job was as a bartender (in his own estimation, a very good one) at Toronto's Royal York Hotel. He conceded that he should have carried through with getting Canadian qualifications in his field; instead, he worked in a variety of retail and other jobs until he started a long-term position with Canada Post. He retired in 2013. He and his wife (also from India) raised four children. When Tariq and I met, he had three grandchildren living in the United States.

Anika was born and raised in Sri Lanka. When we met, she was seventy-two. She had come to Canada with her husband and two children more than thirty years earlier, to escape Sri Lanka's bitter civil unrest. She considered herself lucky to have got an office job in a friendly Italian company, where she worked for more than twenty years, until her retirement at sixty-nine.

Mike, seventy-four when we met, was the only child of a single mother who was determined to keep him busy and out of mischief. She bought him a membership to the Winnipeg YMCA. His involvement in its programs, from a very young age, launched him on a long career in recreation management.

Angela lived all her life in Vancouver. She did office work until her retirement in 2013. She also raised two children as a single mother, and there were struggles along the way. When we met, she was seventy-one, and life was much better. She had three grandchildren, to whom she was devoted and whose presence in her life influenced some of her volunteering. All her family (siblings, too) lived nearby, and she was still in touch with friends she had known since preschool. There was also a new partner in the picture.

All the stories I heard included turning points. Life intervened in surprising or happy or tragic ways to send people in directions they could never have predicted. Happy interventions included meetings with people who turned out to be life-long partners, or side interests that turned into meaningful work. But I also heard about early illnesses, life-changing accidents, financial stresses, relationship breakdowns, the death of partners, and the death of children.

A life-course perspective helped me understand how people's present circumstances had been shaped by what had gone before. As other researchers discovered, privilege tended to play forward, just as disadvantage did. Cynthia's situation (described in the Introduction) was one example. It was echoed by Leslie. She was sixty-three when we first spoke, and living on a disability pension in subsidized housing. Leslie was adopted, and her family connections broke down as she grew up – partly because family members didn't accept that she was lesbian. She started but didn't finish nurse training and spent most of her working life as a personal support worker, until an accident forced her into early retirement at fifty-nine. (She was one of those baby-boom workers whose working life was unstable.)

In addition to her living situation, and her poor health, Leslie had no surviving family and few friends. Her situation was, in a word, precarious. In fact, by 2019 there was a growing recognition among gerontologists that *precarity* accurately characterized the aging process for many vulnerable groups – including those living in poverty. In the case of Cynthia and Leslie, precarity was made even more acute by the absence of social support.

In all the stories I heard, I came to appreciate, again and again, the power of our connection to people. The life-course principle of linked lives was one way to think about this. And there were other helpful perspectives. For example, another feature of family (and other) connections is that we tend to carry them with us as we (and they) age. Researchers call this the *convoy* model of aging. Who is in our convoys as we age determines the social ties we can call on for emotional, and practical, support.

The convoy model builds on work by sociologist Mark Granovetter, whose 1973 study, "The Strength of Weak Ties," has had a lasting impact on researchers' thinking about social ties. He distinguishes between strong ties (close, intimate friendships) and weak ties (distant or more instrumental). His point is that we need both – dear family members and good friends who sustain us emotionally, and a range of other people to connect us to the wider world.

Our lives are embedded in relationships with people. People are at the heart of our experience of aging and our thinking about getting even older. All the people I spoke with helped me to see this clearly.

2

Family Matters

We know that front-wave boomers come with a history – partly, from the *life course perspective* described in the previous chapter, the result of their passage through a particular historical period, partly based on the individual choices they made and the particular paths they followed along the way.

But we also need to take their present circumstances into account by acknowledging the relationships in which they are embedded, the lives to which theirs are linked – in short, the social convoys they are travelling with.

For most people, families are places where social convoys start to be built. We carry them with us as we (and the people in them) age. Over time, these convoys change, and they usually grow. Of all the people I spoke with, few illustrated this growth and change more clearly than Larry and Jennifer.

Thirty-some years ago, when they were looking to settle down and buy a home not too far from Toronto, Larry's father and stepmother had a suggestion. They were snowbirds who spent half their time in the United States. They wanted a Canadian home base, and they also wanted to support Larry and Jennifer. A duplex arrangement in which Larry's father and stepmother would be paying tenants seemed like a good option. Larry and Jennifer agreed. They bought a two-level duplex in Burlington and moved into the ground-floor unit. Larry's parents, when they were around, lived upstairs. In time, two generations became three when Larry and Jennifer's two children arrived.

The most remarkable thing about this arrangement was how long it lasted. With some modifications, it was still in place in October 2019, when Larry, Jennifer, and I got in touch. In the early years, the grandparents gave loving attention to the grandchildren (who also spent time with them at their US home during the summer). The joint homes became a family hub for close-knit siblings on both sides of the family. Over time, things changed. Bill, the grandfather, ninety at the time of that first conversation, was in generally good health and spirits but slowly losing his short-term memory. He needed more care, and Larry and Jennifer were working with his eighty-year-old wife, Helen, to provide it. Five years earlier, Larry had renovated the downstairs unit to make it more age-friendly; Bill and Helen moved downstairs, and Larry and Jennifer moved upstairs. Larry did all the chores and a lot of the cooking. The plan was to care for Bill and Helen at home for as long as possible.

Larry and Jennifer were then sixty-three and sixty-five. The multigenerational model they established had enduring effects. Their daughter, married with a new baby, lived in the same community. She announced that she and her husband would "have dibs on" the care of Larry and Jennifer when they got older. Their son lived in Vancouver but said he'd be happy to move back to the neighbourhood in the future.

Though this multigenerational model of family life and care is common in immigrant and Indigenous communities, among Canadian families overall, it is rare. As Larry and Jennifer described it, it was an unusual but very happy situation. "It may seem special to other people, but we've been living this for thirty years now," Larry said.

It was not just the living arrangements that made this a special story. Other family members lived in close geographic proximity, and the siblings, as well as children and grandchildren, were close emotionally. Jennifer remarked: "I'm always astounded when I hear people that don't speak to their siblings. It's so foreign to me. I don't get it." Finally, although it was Larry's second marriage, he and Jennifer had been together for more than thirty years.

Their situation was noteworthy because it was no longer representative of family life for many older baby boomers. Though a high proportion of Canadians in this age group had children, there was no guarantee that their children would be close at hand as adults. The realities of a globalizing economy made it likely that they would move to work and establish families elsewhere. That's assuming, of course, that they established families in the first place. As the previous chapter also noted, the millennial offspring of the baby boomer cohort are delaying having children, if they have them at all. If they have them, they are having fewer than their forebears did. Grandparenthood for many boomers might be delayed, or off the table. Then there was the significant minority of front-wave boomers who had neither children nor grandchildren – and the number, with or without children, who didn't have partners. All of this suggested a huge diversity of family contexts. There might or might not be children, or grandchildren, who might or might not live close at hand. Multi-generational connections, partner relationships, and other family ties were similarly varied. And all this said nothing of the *quality* of the relationships.

So the question of who counted as family for this group was a big one. It was exactly the question sociologist Ingrid Connidis, an eminent Canadian scholar of aging, has also asked. Connidis suggests that *count* could be understood in three ways. It could be a tally – literally, the number of people in the family group (however *family* was understood.) It could refer to who *mattered*, which relationships were meaningful to people. It could also mean people who could be counted on. Connidis writes: "Asking who can be counted on raises the issue of which family members older people can rely on when they need support – who will help when help is needed. For old and young alike, the corollary to the question, Who can I count on?, is the question, Will someone need to count on me?" Diverse family contexts and differences in who counted appeared in the many family stories I heard, and in others I learned about along the way. I pursued these stories because – when you want to know, as I did, who was in people's lives and, ultimately, who could be counted on – families were a good place to start. I began with the stories closest to home.

IN 2016, ACCORDING TO survey data, about two-thirds of Canadians over sixty-five were married or living in common-law relationships. This was also the case for more than half the people I spoke with, but their stories reflected an amazing range of experiences.

At the time of our first conversation, Gary was seventy-five and had been married for some fifty-five years. His relationship with his wife was one of enduring devotion, and clearly the most significant connection in his life. It showed in his descriptions of how they spent their time, from mornings working on their independent projects to dinner and relaxing in front of the TV. "We've been very happy," he said. He went on to tell a story about the TV watching that said it all:

> At one point, we thought, well, we'll get a couple of these [La-Z-Boy] big chairs. And we had them for a while. And we said one day, "Like, this isn't right." And we went back to a loveseat because, with chairs, it was too separate. We went back to the two-seat loveseat in front of the TV ... It felt more comfortable.

James had a story in a similar vein. He and his wife had just celebrated their fortieth wedding anniversary with a two-week cruise. They did a lot together. And though there were occasional differences, they were not enough to be disruptive. "We just compromise, and find a middle path," James said. Penny jokingly described herself as a "child bride." She and her husband married when she was twenty-one. When we talked, forty-nine years later, she spoke of their life together and his support through the moves they had made, internationally and across Canada, during her career. Fahad, aged sixty-eight when we met, came to Canada from Pakistan when he was twelve. His arranged marriage (during a trip to Pakistan in his late twenties) had lasted for nearly forty years.

There were many other stories of long-term (and hopefully happy) marriages, but these were rarely first marriages. Marital breakdowns and divorce followed by longer-lasting second (or occasionally third) marriages were common. In fact, the boomer generation's tumultuous marriage history was certainly represented.

At the time of our first conversation, Anne and Donald had been married for thirty-one years. It was Anne's second marriage. Her first, when she was in her early twenties, ended after thirteen years. Four years later, she met Donald through his brother, a work colleague. They went on a blind date – and married a year later. Canadian-born Paul went to university in Oregon, where he worked and got married. The marriage was short-lived; he separated from his first wife and returned to Canada. When we met, he and his second wife had been married forty years.

Marriage and relationship stories also varied among older baby boomers who were gay and lesbian. For one thing, they couldn't marry legally till 2005, when most would have been in their fifties. That, of course, did not prevent the formation of long-lasting relationships – like the one described by Matthieu. Before we spoke, he forwarded a newspaper story published the previous Valentine's Day; it described his meeting with his partner – they were both on the rebound from earlier relationships – in a Montreal bar. Though there had been changes over time, the relationship had lasted forty-seven years.

Given the far less tolerant era in which this group came of age, it was not surprising to hear about heterosexual first relationships (often marriages, with children) that ended when one or the other partner came out. Kurt got married when he was twenty, his wife nineteen. "It seems impossible now, looking back at it," he said. "We were children." The marriage lasted for twenty-eight years and, Kurt said, "It wasn't bad – like any other marriage, it had highs and lows." It ended when his wife, after a crisis at work and some "heavy-duty counselling," recognized she was lesbian. Both remarried. Kurt and his second wife had now been together for more than twenty years.

Keith had his own story of coming out. He'd also married young, and he and his wife had three children. It was years later, when he was in his forties, that things changed. As he put it, "I started to deal with the sexual-identity issues." That led to the breakup of the marriage three years later. When we spoke, many more years after that, Keith was in a long-term and happy gay relationship.

Not all divorces or relationship breakdowns led to new relationships. Many in the group had been single a long time. And their rates of divorce and remarriage reflected statistics, in Canada and elsewhere, showing that divorce rates increase with age – and that men are more likely than women to remarry. I also found examples of another emerging relationship category – couples who share an intimate relationship but do not live together (known as LATs, or "living apart together"). Researchers, in fact, are starting to recognize these types of relationships as being of particular interest to aging adults. Today's front-wave boomers came of age during the sexual revolution of the 1960s, and growing numbers of them were divorced by the time they entered old age. Most are not interested in remarrying – and this is particularly true of women. As LAT couples, they are participating in another kind of sexual revolution.

Sociologists Laura Funk and Karen Kobayashi studied LAT couples in Victoria and Vancouver to explore their preference for living apart. One of their interviewees, who grew up in the 1960s, concurred that her generation might be "a little bit more independent thinking." Others spoke of valuing independence and protecting the relationship from the stresses that inevitably arise when people live together. Gender played a role. Women spoke of reaching the point where they wanted control over their lives; they wanted to be in a position of not having to care for others. As one woman put it: "I think a lot of women feel like I do when they get to this stage. The kids are grown. Your parents aren't sick ... For once in your life, it's just about you." This view was also expressed in a 2019 *Globe and Mail* article tellingly headlined "The New Reality of Dating over 65: Men Want to Live Together, Women Don't."

Others lived together but in common-law relationships. And some of these relationships were relatively new. Sarah, at sixty-eight, had been divorced and on her own for ten years before meeting a new partner. When we met, they had been together for eight years and living together for three. Mel, at sixty-five, was widowed for many years before meeting his current partner in 2010. He told me they had "a committed life-long partnership." But he also spoke of the challenges of "putting people in their sixties together." People get set in their ways, he said. "It's one of the harder things I've had to do."

Several had divorced later in life, and women were the more frequent initiators. Emma was in her sixties when she divorced her husband after thirty-two years of marriage. Her decision came after a big trip abroad that ended with a visit with her parents in England. Then in their nineties, her parents had been married some seventy years. She found herself confronting a similar prospect and had an epiphany: "I realized on this trip, I couldn't live with this man for another thirty years." It was a difficult decision ("he's not a bad man"), one she acknowledged was much harder on her husband ("he had no idea"). But it was the start of a new life for her.

Bruce was sixty-eight when we first spoke. He had been separated for three years after a thirty-seven-year marriage. The director of a national nonprofit organization, he saw the separation, instigated by his wife, as one of the costs of his demanding job. "It was more her than anything else," he said. "The way she describes it is, she wanted to have a relationship with somebody, and she can't have it with me because I'm married to [the organization]." Bruce, like Emma, faced a future without a partner. But both had children. That was the case for most people in the group, whether partnered or single. As parents, and often as grandparents, too, their family circles were potentially powerful sources for relationships across the generations.

BOTH BRUCE AND EMMA also had surviving parents, so (as with Larry and Jennifer) there was an extra level to their intergenerational ties. Emma's parents, as just noted, were in their nineties and lived in England. So part of Emma's family work involved phone calls and frequent visits (coordinated with her sister, who also lived outside the United Kingdom).

When we first spoke, Bruce's mother was a remarkably independent ninety-year-old who lived in the same community as Bruce and his two sisters. All family members kept in close touch. In addition to having three children, Bruce also had two grandchildren; like Larry and Jennifer, he was part of a closely connected four-generation family. He left work early once a week to pick up one of the grandchildren from the school bus. Together, they often went to visit his mother.

Larry and Jennifer's experience of multigenerational housing was rare in demographic terms but certainly not unknown among the people I spoke with. Two of Joyce's children immigrated to Canada from Barbados. Her son sponsored her to live with his family – including his nine-year-old son – in 2013. In exchange for the dependence on her son that the federal sponsorship program demanded, she helped care for her grandson and support his working parents.

When civil unrest in Sri Lanka accelerated in the early 1990s, Anika sponsored her (long-widowed) mother. The arrangement lasted for twenty-two years – almost until her mother's death. Anika's children were still in school when their grandmother arrived, and the parents worked. Anika said she was "a great help." Grace's mother lived with Grace and her three children for the last twenty years of her life; she was, in Grace's words, "a great grandmother."

For Anika and Grace, coresidence with aging parents was in the past but remembered with gratitude and love. I also spoke with people who were part of the "sandwich generation" – still caring for their parents and also offering support to children and grandchildren. Larry and Jennifer were good examples. But whereas they cared for one cheerful and lovable ninety-year-old at home, and enjoyed just one young grandson, Ruth's situation was much more complicated.

At sixty-eight, married and living in southern Ontario, Ruth was the mother of four daughters and grandmother of thirteen grandchildren. She'd spent the past twenty years caring for aging parents. Her mother had died four years earlier, but her ninety-three-year-old father, suffering from dementia, was very much part of her life. Though he did not live with her, and though there was a network of paid caregivers to supplement the resources of the private retirement home where he lived, she said the job of overseeing his care took "a humongous amount" of her time. (The quality of his care was an ongoing concern. The day we first talked, she had visited him in the morning and noticed he hadn't been shaved. So she shaved him.)

Two of Ruth's daughters and seven grandchildren lived locally. She and her husband took care of the younger ones two evenings a week, and that care included homework help (all had learning challenges). They also drove the kids around, fixed dinner for both families every couple of weeks, and helped hold "cousin camp" for the three Ontario daughters and their eleven children every Thanksgiving. Friends and relatives often came to stay over the summer.

Ruth also had a time-consuming leadership position in her church. "I really never thought I would get to be my age and as busy as I am," she said. In an email exchange, she noted that she had been "very tired" recently. "I think that it's because I have been so involved."

Other people's experiences of multigenerational family life were less complex than Ruth's because their aging parents didn't live close by or were less in need of care. Sometimes, other family members, mainly siblings, could step in. It's worth noting, though, that sibling relationships could also be strained by the negotiations that surround family support. Ruth, in fact, had a sister who helped with their father's care. She reported that her sister was "great to work with" and that they got along "really well." But, she added, "She will be doing a lot of travelling this coming winter, which leaves all of Dad's care to me."

Ingrid Connidis and sociologist Candace Kemp studied ten multi-generational Canadian families to explore how these sibling negotiations take place. In one case, negotiations involved three daughters aged sixty-nine, sixty-seven, and fifty-seven over the care of their eighty-nine-year-old father, who lived with the eldest daughter, Mary. Mary observed that her sisters were her family, but she was "not involved in their lives, really, except where [their] parents are concerned." The second sister, Beth, said of the others, "Well, we're friends, but we hardly ever see each other." (A fourth sister did not participate in the study or her father's care. She lived an hour away and spent part of the winters in Arizona.)

When her father refused to go into institutional care – the sisters' preferred option – Mary agreed to have him live with her because she was divorced, retired, and living alone. It seemed the obvious choice. This move followed years when Beth had supported him in his home. But the sense was that legitimate excuses (like other work or family responsibilities) were deployed to relieve siblings from sharing in his care. Connidis and Kemp note: "There were few efforts to share filial responsibility in an equitable manner. The ... sisters tend to see caring for their father as a default position; support is offered if no one else can do it or can be 'conned' into doing it."

The broader message is that sometimes it's hard to share support. Excuses might be legitimate. Aging baby boomers such as Ruth, Mary, and Beth took turns providing care to aging parents. But the time might come when their children will be called on to support *them* – and those negotiations might not be easy. Connidis and Kemp comment:

> The reality of an aging population and changing families means that siblings may find themselves willing, yet unable to negotiate providing all of the support that their parents need. More divorce, more parents-in-law, more step-parents, fewer children, greater longevity, and varying views among old people will make such a scenario increasingly common.

In my 2019 conversations, however, I heard more about intergenerational support going in the opposite direction – not to boomers' aging parents but to their children, usually in the form of support for grandchildren. Ruth's care of her grandchildren was a case in point. Sarah was another good example. At sixty-eight and recently retired in Edmonton, she was the mother of two daughters who lived close by – and who, between them, had three children under three. Providing child care and meals, along with plenty of moral support through daily texts and phone calls, took up a lot of her time. In Calgary, seventy-four-year-old Mike's daughter used his home office to run her business. Her two-year-old came with her almost every day, and Mike and his wife were very engaged in his care.

In Winnipeg, seventy-one-year-old Katie and her husband shared the care of their son's two boys with the boys' other grandfather. The arrangement developed to avoid the need for paid daycare when their daughter-in-law returned to part-time work. It amounted to about one day a week. "It's lovely to have the time with them, just by ourselves," Katie said. They had another son who lived with his wife and son in Calgary. They visited him every three months or so. Between visits, they connected by FaceTime and sent gift parcels.

In Saint John, Leanne, at sixty-five, described herself as a "bicoastal grandmother" because she had one daughter in Saint John and another in Vancouver. She had two teenage grandchildren close to home and a seven-year-old and a two-year-old in Vancouver. She had been retired for five years, and spent time driving her fourteen-year-old granddaughter and her friends around and sending messages to her seventeen-year-old grandson, who had a summer job.

Like Katie, she wanted to stay close to the more distant family members in Vancouver. Long divorced, she could make her own decisions about where she would spend her time. With careful money management, she was able to spend extended periods in Vancouver – usually six or seven weeks at a time – a couple of times a year.

I found that single grandfathers were also active participants in their grandchildren's lives. In Toronto, seventy-five-year-old Patrick took the eldest of his three grandchildren to karate twice a week. Bruce had a similar weekly commitment.

Geographical distance shaped family connections in interesting ways. If people had young grandchildren who lived far away, extended visits (like Leanne's trips to Vancouver) proved to be the best way to stay close for those able to afford them. If people had older grandchildren, sometimes the children visited them. Bina, a sixty-seven-year-old widow in Calgary, had grandchildren both close at hand and far away – in her case in Calgary and Toronto. She picked up her Calgary grandchildren from school once a week and fed and entertained them. During spring break, and for a month in the summer, she visited her two Toronto grandchildren to help out while their parents worked. Also in the summer, she brought the Toronto grandchildren back with her to spend a month in Calgary so they could get to know their cousins.

Those demographic shifts noted earlier were also reflected in relationships with grandchildren whose ages varied widely. Whereas Mike at seventy-four enjoyed regular visits from his two-year-old grandson, seventy-six-year-old Richard spoke of FaceTime chats with his nineteen-year-old grandson away at university. Gary and his wife also had adult grandchildren; at seventy-five, Gary was about to become a great-grandfather.

With or without grandchildren, people's in-person contact with their adult children varied, and here, too, relative proximity played a role. Nicole and her husband, in Edmonton, represented one end of a contact continuum. Their three sons also lived in Edmonton – as Nicole put it, within cycling distance of their parents. All were partnered, had professional jobs, and were unlikely to move away. There was a lot of family interaction, including weekly dinners. Grandchildren in the future were a strong possibility.

Christine, in Vancouver, exemplified the other end of the contact continuum, with one son in Australia. Grace, in Victoria, had two sons, one in Saskatoon and one in the United Kingdom. Many parents had children who lived in other provinces, too far away for frequent visits. In most cases, there *were* visits – sometimes subsidized by children better positioned to afford airfares. And most parents were comfortable using online meeting options. Christine and Grace had joined the legion of transnational families who depended on information and communications technologies to stay close.

Their experiences matched the findings of sociologist Loretta Baldassar, who has spent years studying intergenerational relationships and caregiving in families separated by distance. How family members manage to "be there" while not being actually present is at the heart of the research; technology, she discovered, has become a means to achieve "co-presence across distance."

Her research includes a wonderful case study that traces the complex means by which one family managed to stay in touch and give support. The family included an elderly widowed mother in an Italian city and her three children, each with their own families in, respectively, another Italian city, Ireland, and Australia. They communicated via multifamily Skype sessions on Sundays, daily phone calls between the mother and her daughter in Italy, text messages among the siblings, and a family WhatsApp chat started when the mother had a stroke.

Baldassar acknowledges that while "being there" in the actual, physical sense is considered preferable to digital communication, the latter should not be underestimated, especially when there are intermittent in-person visits as well. Although not all transnational families have the resources to make use of new technologies in this way, the case study shows how communications technologies can deepen bonds and mutual support between people separated by distance.

NOT SURPRISINGLY, GIVEN THE complex marital histories of front-wave boomers, many of the people I spoke with also had relationships with stepchildren and step-grandchildren. As research in the area shows, these relationships can be complicated.

Brenda and Ursula, for example, were stepmothers in families where their stepchildren's biological father had died. Brenda said she was "very good friends" with her stepchildren but found there was "one degree of separation" because of their closeness to their biological mother. Ursula had married for the first time at forty-five. Her husband had two sons, aged nine and eleven at the time. Some four years before we spoke, and after nearly twenty years of marriage, Ursula's husband died of a massive stroke. What followed was "a very dark period" in which there was little contact with her stepsons – who, she realized, were also grieving. But that too changed over time. The elder son and his partner were with her when she had to put the beloved family dog down. Recently, she said she was "totally blown away" when he called her: "He said, 'I want to talk to you because I want your blessing, because I want to ask [partner] to marry me.'" She told him how moved she was that he had thought to include her in his plans. "I was blubbering!" she said. He responded, "Well, you're part of this, too, you know."

Some of the step-parent relationships I heard about were as warm and mutually supportive as connections with biological children could be. Doug met his second wife in 1982. Her son was eight when they married and, according to Doug, thought of him as his dad. When Doug and I first spoke, the stepson and his family lived about an hour away, and the family connections were close.

In Walt's case, his second wife, Jane, had also been married before. Both had adult children. They continued to be involved with their own children, but there was plenty of crossover. When Walt and I met, the two were providing meals monthly to busy daughters with children on both sides of the family.

In addition to being step-parents, Walt and Jane were also step-grandparents, a role and relationship of increasing interest to researchers, especially when the step-grandparent joins the family when the grandchildren are quite young. In one study, two-thirds of the step-grandchildren felt their step-grandparents were important kin, either because they'd replaced absent biological grandparents or because they were emotionally present alongside actively engaged biological grandparents. One-third found their step-grandparents emotionally distant. These perceptions seemed to be shaped by their parents' relationships with the step-grandparents. If the two older generations had warm, familial relationships, the connections between step-grandchildren and step-grandparents were likely to be the same.

Patrick's case offers another angle on relationships in complicated blended families. Widowed when his two sons were five and three, Patrick remarried about two and a half years later. After about ten years, he and his second wife had two daughters, two years apart. The older boys were then nineteen and seventeen. They were immediately taken with the babies. In Patrick's words, two "smelly teenage boys" learned something about nurturing – "which was phenomenal for them, and for us." It was "a total love affair, between my two sons and my two daughters, that lasted, and still lasts today." When Patrick and I met, his daughters were in their early twenties, and the older of his two sons was married with three children of his own.

THERE WAS PLENTY OF EVIDENCE, in many of the stories I heard, that family relationships had their ups and downs. Two categories of parent–adult-child relationships stood out. The first included families in which adult children needed support.

In Denise's case, when her daughter's marriage broke up, she and her husband took her and her children in. Mark and his wife provided a home for his stepson, who was dealing with clinical depression. Angela, too, was helping her daughter deal with a cancer diagnosis. In an email, she wrote:

> I have been busy with her mostly attending appointments so I could grasp what they were telling her. She would listen but not hear which is very typical when you are receiving news that you don't want. This whole experience has left me feeling helpless and worried. As a mom you are supposed to be able to come to the rescue and I can't make it better for her.

When we were last in touch, Angela's daughter was doing well, Denise's daughter and family had moved on, and Mark was expecting the same of his stepson.

But sometimes demands on aging parents never end. Parents of children with disabilities have ongoing responsibilities, and worries. Estimates of the number of parents in this situation are hard to come by, but recent studies suggest that there are many challenges, regardless of whether the children live with their parents. And challenges loom ever larger as both parents and children age.

Fiona and Jim knew all about the challenges. Aged seventy-one and seventy-six, they had a forty-seven-year-old son, Trevor, who had several severe disabilities. He was blind due to a genetic disorder. He was also autistic, did not speak, and had other behavioural issues. He'd lived in community settings since he was eighteen, but the management of his care had been stressful and time-consuming, especially for Fiona. Finding, and retaining, care workers had been a big part of the problem – though when we spoke they had a team in place they trusted. They had no other family support, and the severity of Trevor's challenges isolated them even from other parents of children with disabilities. They hoped to find a place for Trevor in a home for seniors with disabilities when he reached the qualifying age of fifty. Jim commented: "The reason we want to do it earlier is that we're not going to be here that long."

Parents' responses are also shaped by family context, the nature of the disability, and perhaps cultural influences as well. Deepak, seventy-three years old, had an autistic son who lived with him and his wife. Seventy-one-year-old Tariq likewise looked after his disabled daughter – though, in that case, she was one of four children, and he had considerable family support. Tariq was retired, but his much younger wife still worked. Their daughter loved to cook; in Tariq's eyes, she was making a valuable contribution to the household. He was sure that if he were to die, both his wife and daughter would be well cared for.

The second category of parent-child relationships that stood out involved front-wave boomers who were coping with uneasy, fragile, or broken relationships with their adult children. Researchers now recognize that many family relationships are *ambivalent* – characterized by both positive and negative feelings. That would not be news to families in general, and to several people I spoke with. "They have busy lives" was a line I heard many times from front-wave boomers reluctant to push for more contact with their adult children. (The busy lives of working adults with young children is also well documented, and a story in itself.)

Sometimes, there seemed to be more to the story. Laura's daughter lived abroad, so in-person contact would have been difficult. But they were not in touch much virtually either. Laura pointed to her daughter's busyness. "I don't want to layer guilt on her," she said. "Nobody needs that crap." She also commented that the daughter had "an anxiety problem" and was sometimes hard to be with.

James's thirty-nine-year-old daughter lived within easy driving distance. He described her as "a bit volatile." On the day we first spoke, James and his wife were going to see her, and her two children, for the first time in several months. "We'll see how it works out," he said. Teresa, in southern Ontario, spoke of a daughter (also an easy drive away) who seldom called and a son in New Brunswick who was often away for work and always busy when home. "The one I can really talk to and vent to is my middle son," she said. "He's in Calgary, and he can cheer me up in, like, two minutes."

In rare cases, relationships had broken down completely, for reasons that weren't always clear (and were probably more complicated than a conversation with a stranger like me could uncover). Sixty-seven-year-old Elizabeth was estranged from both her children. Her younger son who had left home twenty years earlier had substance abuse issues. She told me he texted maybe twice a year. Her older son lived two kilometres away but was not in contact. She didn't have his phone number.

Sometimes, family trauma involving adult children required grandparents to take over the raising of their grandchildren. According to the 2016 census, some thirty-two thousand Canadian children were living in "skipped-generation" families – that is, without their parents present. Author Gary Garrison, himself helping to raise step-grandchildren, suggests the number might be much higher than census counts reveal because grandparents are reluctant to disclose their situation, even on a census form. Grandparents step in when their adult child is unable to parent, for a range of reasons that might include mental or physical health issues, or addiction, or extreme poverty, or imprisonment. While recent statistics are hard to find, Garrison and other sources also note the disproportionate number of Indigenous grandparents caring for their grandchildren in skipped-generation households – a consequence of the multigenerational trauma wrought by residential schools, the Sixties Scoop, and other assaults on traditional Indigenous family life. Garrison's book *Raising Grandkids* is full of poignant stories about pain that crosses three generations and the enormous challenges caregiver grandparents face. As one Indigenous grandmother told researchers, "I never had that childhood connection with my grandparents or my mother, my relatives. I feel it is very important ... my grandchildren need that. And maybe they'll feel more secure than our generation."

Intergenerational reciprocity and support are hard to see in these situations. Grandparents raising grandchildren, for example, seem to be giving much more than they are taking. But the intergenerational family connections are built in. This may not be the case for those who don't have children.

SURVEY DATA SUGGEST THAT about 10 percent of people sixty-five and older in Canada are childless. I assumed, without pressing for answers, that there would be a mix among the people I spoke with of those who had chosen not to have children and those whose childlessness was involuntary. I found examples of both. There were certainly those who had been resolute in their wish not to go the conventional family route. When I asked Hope about her immediate family, she responded firmly, "Single, single, single! By choice, from the beginning. Never wanted children. Never wanted a permanent partner. No, no."

Others responded to circumstances. Penny, the twenty-one-year-old "child bride," had worked in a professional, male-dominated environment with relentless expectations about productivity. She commented: "I never had children, and I think it's just – there never seemed to be a time ... There isn't a right time, in [my work] especially."

Gay men I spoke with had no children unless they'd previously been in a heterosexual relationship. This may have been the outcome of spending their young adulthood in a world (and a country) much less tolerant of gay parenting than it is today. (For example, it wasn't until 2000 that Ontario's Child and Family Services Act was amended to allow for same-sex adoptions.) People such as Matthieu and his partner couldn't have become parents in the conventional sense, even if they had wanted to. "We did discuss it, at some point," he said. "At the time, it would have been very difficult to do, because it would have been revealing a lifestyle that was at the time illegal. By the time that was over, I figured I was a bit too old."

What Matthieu did have, however, were siblings, nieces, and nephews. He was devoted to them, and they were devoted to him. He told the story of a surprise party one of his sisters organized to celebrate the twenty years that Matthieu and his partner had been together. All the siblings, nieces, and nephews were there. His godson and one of his nieces lived with him and his partner while they went to university; a great-nephew also signed up to stay. (Family studies scholar Robert Milardo calls aunts and uncles "the forgotten kin" and notes the important role they play in many families.)

Close connections with nieces and nephews often follow from close connections with siblings. For people without their own children, these can be important relationships. Anne and Donald had no children of their own but enjoyed their ties to Donald's extended family. Anne's beloved brother had died, but she was close to his wife, son, and two-year-old grandson. When Narek lost a brother, he stepped in to be something of a surrogate father to his two nephews.

Some front-wave boomers I spoke with were technically "elder orphans" – living alone, without partners and without children. The term gained some media coverage in Canada based on research by US geriatrician Maria Carney. A 2016 paper by Carney and her colleagues contained a warning that older people in this category were at heightened risk of loneliness and isolation, with potentially serious consequences for their health. There is some disagreement about the term and what it implies. Psychologist Bella DePaulo describes it as inaccurate – orphans are people without parents, not people without children – as well as pitying, stigmatizing, and ageist. Terminology aside, relationships to siblings and their children may be significant for people without partners or children of their own.

Those I spoke with had different experiences in this respect. Thelma lived in Toronto. She had one sister who lived elsewhere in Ontario whom she did not see often. Her nephew and his family, however, lived in the city. He and his partner were her executors, with power of attorney on health issues, and she benefitted from his partner's astute financial advice.

When I spoke with her, Gail had lived solo for twenty-five years following two marriages. Having grown up in an abusive and dysfunctional family, she, too, had chosen not to have children. She speculated: "Could I be a good parent, being raised in the family I was raised in?" Gail's main family connection was with nieces who lived an hour away. She said they loved her as she loved them. She commented that she had much better relationships with them than with her siblings.

In Dave's case, though, it was his siblings who came through when he needed them. At sixty-seven, he was the oldest of three, and had a ninety-three-year-old mother living in a retirement home. He had recently retired from his retail and bookkeeping job. The family was geographically scattered – only Dave lived in Calgary. He told me that when he went through cancer surgery, his brother came to stay overnight when he got home from hospital, and his sister stayed for a week to help him recover. They kept in sporadic contact by phone. He was not in touch with their children.

WE AGING BABY BOOMERS need people to share our lives, people who will be there for us in times of need. It's worth remembering the distinction between family members who *matter,* and those who can be *counted on,* compared to those who just happen to be around. Clearly, there are wide differences in the number and quality of family ties people can draw on, from the rich multigenerational connections available to Larry and Jennifer, to the reduced circle available to people such as Gail or Dave. Their family convoys are quite different; they show, in another way, how privilege and precarity can play out.

Larry and Jennifer's convoy changed over time as its members aged and the family expanded. As their parents reached a new stage of very old age, their convoy also grew to include their children's partners and a grandchild. The benefits of having younger people in the family convoy are easy to see. People like Larry and Jennifer are people who can be counted on. They offer support in two directions – to aging parents and to adult children. In return, they understand that family help will be available to them too.

Dave's family situation is a different story. He is not alone in having few family contacts of any kind in his convoy, and none that can easily offer long-term support. For people like Dave, family relationships are not the ones that will sustain him as he ages. The question of who else is around, who matters, and who can be counted on, would require a broader search.

3

Friends and Communities

One of the people I spoke with was a sixty-nine-year-old retired librarian from Halifax. We talked, among other things, about her extensive postretirement activities. For several years, she had volunteered for an urban farm. She did some physical work but also (because of her extensive organizational experience) participated in core planning. She worked with a team of young people, so there was some mentoring involved too. She played bridge regularly and sang in a drop-in choir. On the day of our conversation, she planned to have lunch with a friend, then go to an aquafit class. She had many friends in her life, both far afield and close at hand. "I meet people for coffee *a lot!*" she said.

The woman was Hope, whose determination to remain single and family-free I describe in the previous chapter. Hope was a so-called elder orphan, but her thriving networks made her lack of family connections seem almost beside the point. Though she didn't want a family in the conventional sense, she intentionally cultivated relationships that were effective alternatives.

When we were first in touch, she lived in an apartment in a house owned by a couple who were old friends. She had known one of the partners for nearly fifty years. "That's as much of a family relationship as I have, and it's as much as I want," she said. They were the people she'd likely call first in an emergency, and they had her power of attorney. But she could think of many other people (fifteen or so, she figured) that she could also call on for support. (They could call her too. She'd recently responded to three emergencies involving a friend with heart problems.)

Her volunteer work put her in almost constant contact with young people, and she felt strongly about the need for intergenerational connections. "I think this is a hugely important question," she said. "When you stop work, and if your kids, if you have kids, aren't around – let's say, they're living in other cities – you can lose contact with young people immediately. And I think it's a problem ... You need young people to just push you out of your comfort zone."

Hope's story certainly challenges the negative implications of being an elder orphan – implications that others have also criticized. Her circumstances also illuminate many of the issues relating to social connections for front-wave boomers. Where she lived, how she spent her time, and who she spent it with are all part of the bigger picture of social connection that I wanted to explore. How did social ties outside of family shape people's social convoys? Would the same diversity, and the sharply contrasting experiences of privilege and precarity evident in other dimensions of boomers' lives, be apparent here too?

It's reasonable to think that in the case of Hope, and other single people without children, connections outside of family would take on extra significance. But many of those with close family connections also knew their social networks needed to be broader. Amy, at sixty-nine, was married and living in Calgary. She had three children (one of them also in Calgary) and six grandchildren. She described her children as busy people. "They have their lives," she said. "There has to be that relationship ... that allows the comfort that they're there, but not a dependency." Amy was well aware of the importance of reaching beyond her family circle. "It isn't family or nothing," she said.

So where, outside of families, do front-wave boomers find their people? And who, of the people they have found, are the people who *matter?* Who are the people, outside of families, who make up their convoys? The answers to these questions, not surprisingly, are rich and complicated. They are also mostly about in-person connections.

It was clear from my conversations – indeed, from the way these conversations were set up – that front-wave boomers were comfortable with information and communications technology. (According to a 2018 Statistics Canada report, 81 percent of people aged sixty-five to seventy-four were online by 2016.) Email was routine, and (judging from some of the material I was sent) occasionally incorporated networks of friends. Facebook came up in some conversations, and those with distant family members were usually proficient with platforms such as FaceTime or Skype. I thought this would be the case for most of the others too.

Support for this conclusion comes in part from work done as far back as 2013 and 2014 in the East York region of Toronto, by researchers interested in older people's social networks and the extent to which they use digital media. The researchers found that "the great majority of East Yorkers" integrated digital media into their everyday lives. More recent studies confirmed this proficiency among older adults. But my conversations suggested that in-person connections were the ones to focus on.

IN-PERSON CONNECTIONS were sometimes close to home – in Hope's case, just upstairs. Bonnie lived technically alone in a self-contained unit in one of British Columbia's well-established cohousing communities. But hers was one of nineteen households linked by a collective commitment to social connectedness and mutual support. In this sense, both she and Hope reinforced the findings of a recent Canadian study showing that older adults living alone – some 25 percent of people over sixty-five, according to the latest census – did not, in fact, seem to be more socially disconnected than those in other living arrangements. *Alone* did not always mean isolated or lonely.

Bonnie's independence within a community was also true of the people I spoke with who had moved to retirement communities. James commented that he and his wife made the move despite the community's clubhouse, which was central to its social life. But they were soon converts; they regularly attended dances and exercise classes and made some friends. "That was an unexpected benefit," he said.

Sharing accommodation was another means of having people around. When I spoke with Helen, she was single and lived in a small town in southern Ontario. She had a daughter and granddaughter in Yukon. Nearly seventy, she had no financial resources beyond her government pensions. She was renting a room in a house with a multi-generational family – grandparents, parents, and a three-year-old. Relationships in the household seemed warm and friendly. The little one came to visit Helen every morning.

Narek at seventy was in a "living apart together" situation with his partner, but he didn't live alone. His house in Vancouver had a suite that he rented out, and he had other tenants, including, for a while, a young man who was aging out of foster care. Diana, in Edmonton, rented rooms in her spacious house to international graduate students. They looked after themselves, but there was some sociability as well. She showed me a video clip of a group get-together that involved dancing in her kitchen. "At the moment, I've got a nice gang," she said.

Several of the people I spoke with had homes in neighbourhoods in which they – and their neighbours – had lived for decades. These neighbourhoods, occupied by aging empty nesters in original family homes, have been given a name – naturally occurring retirement communities, or NORCs. Along with the label has come recognition, by scholars of aging as well as advocates and residents, that with careful design and resource planning, NORCs might be places where

older people could stay in their homes for the long haul, a phenomenon now called "aging in place."

Amy lived in a Calgary NORC, and in fact, when we met, work
was underway to build up social connections – like the occasional pub
nights, regular men's coffee group meetings, and other activities – to
make it just the sort of community that would allow aging in place.

Katie, in Winnipeg, also lived in what sounded very much like
a NORC. She and her husband had raised their children there and
had been in the same house for some thirty years. Among her
other connections, Katie belonged to a long-standing neighbourhood
book club.

In almost every case, home and neighbourhood connections
were not the only ones that mattered, as Hope's story clearly illus-
trates. Katie said she was close to her neighbours, but as a retired
teacher, she belonged to another book club with colleagues from her
last school. She was also a member of an educators' sorority that had
many young women members. And she was involved in social justice
and other work with her church community (not to mention the
child care she and her husband provided to their grandchildren). "I
love people," she said.

Personal interests and social commitments were behind many of
the connections people made outside their families. Gary sang in a
men's choir and was president of the woodshop in his retirement
community. Dan had recently retired from a federal government job
and lived alone in Ottawa. He was a self-described "consummate
introvert" – and a passionate cat lover – so he volunteered weekly
at the local Humane Society.

Angela's twin grandchildren were born prematurely and were in
a hospital neonatal intensive care unit for a time. Moved and motivated by that experience, she became a volunteer in the unit, giving
support to families. Later, she became a busy school volunteer. Geoff,
in Ottawa, and Rod, in Calgary, were both active as volunteers in
their cities' LGBTQ2S+ support organizations.

Paul and his wife did not have children or grandchildren but were involved in a volunteer grandparents' group in their BC community. Beyond that, though, Paul's circle was wide. He had friends among his neighbours and others who were also long-standing (he had a weekly dinner date with one of them). He also took aquafit and dance classes.

Classes were a source of interest and sociability for many. Many are held at local community associations, often particularly targeting older people. Some community centres operate as hubs for a wide range of groups and needs. On one of my visits to Toronto, I was introduced to the Rexdale Community Hub. Its women's centre ran an ethnocultural seniors' program that sometimes hosted classes and activities in the first language of the participants. I discovered an amazingly diverse selection of offerings. Joyce, sponsored by her son to come to Canada from Barbados in 2013, was involved with the African and Caribbean Seniors' Group. Anika came to the centre four times a week for Zumba and yoga classes.

Anika was also an active member of her church, a connection that others also mentioned. Though recent data on Canadians' religious affiliation is hard to come by – particularly active participation in religious communities – what seems clear is that older people are more likely to be involved. And their involvement tends to be sociable as well as spiritual.

When Ben retired, he and his wife moved to Hamilton to be closer to a daughter living in Toronto. They knew ahead of time that it would be important to be involved in their local synagogue. "It's not that we're very religious," he said. It was rather that the synagogue would be a "base of operations," a way to become connected. That's what happened. "The synagogue became the centre of our life," he said. Over time, they took up service work – Ben became a member of the synagogue's board, and both he and his wife were choir members. But the social side was key. They had other, old friends in their lives, but following their move, all their friendships were through the synagogue. I asked if these were the people they'd call in an emergency. "Not that we would exclude others, but friends we would call up are synagogue friends," he said.

Walt told a similar story about the role of church in his life. He belonged to a church men's group that had been meeting regularly for some twenty years, and another one, more recently formed, that met weekly. He and his wife also belonged to a home church group and had hosted a meeting the night before we met. In addition to the couple's active family connections, Walt's faith-based relationships constituted the bulk of his nonfamily social ties. "For me, the faith is extremely important," he said. "It provides hope and meaning and purpose and fulfillment and community."

Bina came to Canada from India in 1975 when she was twenty-three. Her multifaceted working life as a librarian gave her a broad range of colleagues and work friends. After she retired, she volunteered in the local food bank and had set up school libraries. Active in her local mosque, she spoke of her Muslim community as the source of her strongest friendships. "I do move, here in Calgary, with my own Muslim friends, seniors," she said. But the connection was not just because they were Muslim. They did have a Koran study, but they also held potlucks. "The food and language and culture, I guess, bring us together that way."

How these sources of connection came together for front-wave boomers was very much an individual matter. People's choices and resources were a wonderful mix. People met in coffee shops and community centres and at the library – and in dog parks too.

I hadn't expected to hear about the ways animals connected their owners to other people. Dog parks, I discovered, were a great social resource. Patrick had lively and ongoing connections with family and friends, but the conversations he had in the dog park became a twice-daily highlight. The dog park itself was pleasantly situated, and he reported that the people he met there were interesting. "It provides community," he said.

Thelma, a so-called elder orphan, had had a career that precluded pet ownership. When she retired, she got a dog. She was less well connected than Patrick, but the dog introduced her to a new community. "I've met a lot of people," she said. "It's a marvellous bridge!" Christopher reported that two of his dog-park contacts became very good friends. They met for coffee at least once a week.

THOSE WITHOUT CHILDREN and grandchildren tend to develop close ties with people the same age. This phenomenon, called *age homophily*, raises the broader question, how do older people meet younger generations? That was the question researchers put to a small group of older people in Ireland, who were identified as having at least one good friend fifteen or more years younger. Their findings were illuminating. For example, despite different contexts, one thing stood out: meetings happened in age-integrated, shared spaces, whether leisure centres, interest groups, former workplaces, or families, spaces where they could meet like-minded people. What brought people together – whether leisure pursuits, hobbies, or interests – acted as a stepping stone to deeper friendships. As they got to know one another, they shared more.

This finding meshed with my own. Hope stressed the importance of intergenerational relationships. Ursula's professional life in music put her in touch with many younger people, including the students she mentored and who helped her too. "I really value that connection," she said. Anne noted the "tons of young knitters" involved in her knitting community. Paul met younger people through his work as an active volunteer grandparent. Other connections were more serendipitous. Christopher reported that his dog park friends were much younger.

Even people with younger family members sought out new intergenerational connections. Karen, who lived in small-town Ontario with four children and a crop of grandchildren, helped run a cooking club for young people as part of a community mentorship program.

Brenda, recently widowed, was thinking about renting a room in her house to a university student. Having been "Mumsy" to many of her daughter's university friends (many of whom were still in touch), she commented, "It's the young ones who I would really like to surround myself with."

Helen spoke of the recent death of her best friend of forty-five years and the failing health of another. But she also had a "fluid" support network across the country, and it was getting younger. "There's only one old crone left in my tight circle," she said. That suited her. Helen estimated that she'd been an activist since she was twelve. She found that conversations with older people tended to involve talking about grandchildren. She wanted to talk about the environment and the state of the world.

Not surprisingly, women seemed to be better connected outside their families than men. Research consistently shows that older men are less likely to participate in community social programming. Especially among older heterosexual couples, men tend to depend on women to organize their social lives. On their own, they are much more likely to be socially isolated.

But I found surprising exceptions. Some of them, like Paul and Patrick, I've already noted. Fahad was another exception. He attended a mosque and described himself as engaged socially in the community (though he wasn't, to use his term, hard-core). He tried to go most Fridays, mostly to meet friends. But his network extended far beyond the mosque. He spoke of annual week-long hiking or kayaking trips with old high school friends and regular lunch get-togethers (for over forty years) with former work colleagues. As a former health care administrator, he was sought out as a teacher and mentor.

John was another volunteer grandparent. He was also in a music community. He played pickleball three or four times a week with his buddies, and he sat on the council of his condominium building. For seven years, he'd been a member of a multi-age men's book club that met monthly at his home.

But these men were unusual. For many, work had been a major focus in their lives, and they found retirement a challenge. They had grown up with social and cultural expectations to be strong and independent – a form of masculinity described as "hegemonic" or socially dominant that is only now showing signs of change.

Several wives spoke about their partners' struggles with life after retirement and speculated on how they'd manage if their wives were not around. As one wife put it: "He would go from the funeral home to a speed dating service, because he could not cope on his own ... It's sad but true. He'd marry the first desperate woman that promised to cook him supper." She was joking, but her assessment of her husband's dependence on her for his social life resonated with other women. "I'm the enabler!" said Amy. "If you were to compare my husband's outreach to mine, I would say mine is [many] times more than his." Anne said, "Sometimes there's a bit of initiation from the bossy wife."

Many of the men I spoke with – men such as Fahad and John, who had no trouble making social connections – recognized the difference in gender expectations. John said he saw it "over and over again." Pierce spoke about it at length, movingly, and from first-hand experience. A university professor retired for ten years, he'd done some part-time teaching until shortly before we met. After a twenty-year marriage and two children, he'd been on his own for several years before meeting his current partner. How were those years on his own? "Awful!" he said. "They were pretty miserable years ... despair, loneliness."

It took a lot of effort to get himself out of that loneliness, and he had good stories of the things he tried (a ballroom dance class was not a successful venture). Happily, thanks to one of the fitness groups he taught, he met his partner. He learned some important lessons along the way, about his need for social connections and the difficulty he (and many other men) had in finding them. He had had close friends. But as a self-described introvert, he'd neglected work-related and other relationships that he could have developed. "I rather regret that now," he said. "If I had to do it over again, there'd be a thousand things I'd do differently."

Thinking more about this, Pierce sent me an email the day after we met. He wrote of the men of his father's generation, often war veterans, who "did not discuss their emotions and were never to show vulnerability." His father had been one of those men. He added: "No wonder so many are unable to have the nurturing and critical relationships that the majority of women have. We men boomers were short-changed and are now impacted for it unless we can break out of our shells around this subject."

One of Pierce's successful outreach attempts came from a lucky encounter – in a local coffee shop – with a men's biking group. He knew one of the members, established that the group met regularly, and asked if he could join. He was looking for other interest groups when we met.

But finding interest groups can be an ongoing challenge. Researchers and men's health advocates have noted a significant lack of community programming targeted at men. The programming that does exist is perceived as being more suited to women. This may be due less to the content of the programs than to the fact women rather than men sign up. Men are noticeably absent from seniors' and community association activities. Social isolation is the risk, if not the result.

Peter is a case in point. When we spoke, he was seventy-seven and had retired (reluctantly) from his manufacturing job five years earlier. "I would not recommend anyone to retire," he said. His wife continued to work, his one volunteer job had ended the year before, and he had a great deal of time on his hands during the day. He filled it with "projects round the house." He also liked to do acrylic painting and was writing his life story. But there were few people around. "My neighbours around here are all retired," he said. "Or, in the wintertime, their houses are empty. They've gone down to Florida, or whatever. And I say to myself, 'I could slip and fall. I could go out in the backyard, I could slip and fall. I could lie there all day' ... There's nobody around to talk to."

ONE OF THE MOST DIRECT attempts in Canada to address this problem, and in the process help end men's social isolation, is the Men's Shed movement. The movement has had a long history in Australia, where the "shed in the back yard" has always been recognized as men's space. By 2019, the movement was also flourishing in the United Kingdom and New Zealand.

The Men's Sheds Canada website recognizes the problem of inviting men to join something that would greatly benefit them, socially and psychologically, without turning off prospective members. It does this with a light, good-humoured touch: "In a shed, men get together for activities like woodworking projects, cooking, bike repairs, music, and yelling at the television during the playoffs." Elsewhere it describes the sheds as a gathering place for men of purpose "and others." They are productive – "maybe." They are places to change the world – "definitely." They offer a helping hand – "you bet." They are *not* a formal training program – "but you may gain some knowledge and skills." They are *not* a health program – "but your health and well-being may improve." They are *not* a service for men – "but you might be of service to others or get advice and support from time to time."

Researchers from the University of Manitoba studied one of the first Canadian men's sheds, in Winnipeg, a few years after its founding in 2010. The men who participated were clear about the advantages of membership. One of them commented: "With all of us living longer and the influx, starting especially from now on of the Baby Boomers, there's going to be a huge need for programming. Many men's social aspects of their lives are run by their spouses ... I believe, men with men contact, it's a different kind of contact, and I think that's very important." Another added: "Being mainly men is very important because men will not talk about some things when there are women around that they will talk to each other when there is not ... I think men will be more open with each other when, when there's not women." The researchers note that while dominant conceptions of masculinity are evident in much of the men's talk, and in the focus on "manly" activities like woodworking, the sheds also provide an environment safe enough for men to be vulnerable and open and, in the process, to build more meaningful relationships with one another.

Several of the men I spoke with were deeply engaged, often as founders or organizers, with men's sheds in Ontario, Manitoba, Alberta, and British Columbia. All of them were strong advocates. "It's like finding religion ... I absolutely and totally believe in it," one commented. These conversations revealed that sheds differed in terms of where they met, how they were organized, and what they offered. In some cases, woodworking was, indeed, a central focus, and local community organizations benefitted from what they produced.

In other cases, the focus was more social. "The centre point of our group is the coffee pot!" one leader commented. He understood the social benefits of working together. "Some of the guys that come to us have been sitting at home for a while," he said. "And so they're kind of bored, and going into a little bit of depression." Health issues can be a common bond. "Busy hands make lips work," he said. "They start talking about it, and then they find that they're not alone with the problem that they have. It so encourages them."

NO MATTER WHAT KIND of social ties might be *available* to people, they still need to do the work of taking them up. For extroverts, this can be easy. Sandra was probably the most socially connected person I spoke with. She and her husband were recently retired, and both did regular volunteer shifts at their local hospital's Ronald McDonald

House. They also played pickleball several times a week, hosted games nights with friends most weekends, and met monthly with a church group. Sandra also had long-term friends in a quilting group.

Others, less well connected, recognized what they might be missing and were intentional about reaching out. Fran, sixty-eight when we spoke, had children and grandchildren close at hand. She also had a husband of thirty-five years who was fifteen years older than she was – a fairly significant gap. Though they still had much in common, the activities they did together had changed, and she was doing more on her own. She had started a book club with three friends. "I can see us building bonds," she said. Realistically, she knew she would likely survive her husband, even though he had longevity in his genes. She and her women friends had been talking for a long time about sharing accommodation, if she did end up alone.

For others, reaching out was harder. When we met, Sarah had recently retired from a busy medical practice that hadn't left much time for a social life. "I had not fostered my friendships when I was working," she said. Like Fran, she had children and grandchildren close by but knew she needed more. When she retired, a "very extroverted" friend got her to join a small women's group. "It's been a huge comfort," she said. "We meet maybe once a month, but [there's] really important talk. We can be very honest with each other." She also reconnected with some former colleagues she hadn't been in touch with for several years who had formed a book club. Sarah knew herself to be an introvert. "I love to be by myself," she said. "But I know that too much is not good. It's kind of like, I need this ... I didn't want to be isolated. I know, [with] my personality, I could be."

Gail understood what Sarah meant. A sixty-eight-year-old retired college instructor, she'd been living alone for some twenty-five years and was in treatment for long-standing depression. She thought it had been about fifteen years since she'd started to isolate herself and friends started to drop away. "And I used to have loads of friends," she said. "I was always the funny one ... I miss me. I miss whoever that person was." She still had one good friend and did one weekly volunteer shift at a charity thrift store, which she enjoyed.

But, otherwise, she had no social life and saw it as "a big need." "I think it's the anxiety that's associated with the depression, that just keeps me, at times, from doing things," she said. She recalled activities, like a book club, that she had enjoyed. "It has caused me to think, 'Get your ass out there' ... start to do some of the things that I *know* I would benefit from, and that I'd like."

Dave had scant family connections and few other social relationships. "It's a little bit of a concern," he said. "Or a wish, I guess, not really a concern, because I've been single all my life. It's not that I really *need* anyone. [But] it would be nice sometimes too." Dave had been retired from his bookkeeping and retail job for two years. "I didn't know what I would do next," he said. "I still really don't." But one thing he was trying out was a local Men's Shed.

IT'S CLEAR THAT THE SOCIAL ties people choose are dependent on tastes and, to quote Sarah, personalities too. But some conversations revealed that social isolation might be imposed, rather than chosen, a consequence of specific circumstances or social barriers.

Through the Rexdale Community Hub ethnocultural seniors' program, I met several participants, actively engaged themselves, who spoke with concern about older at-risk immigrants in the community. Notable among them were those who had been sponsored by their adult children; they were often financially dependent, had limited English, lived in busy and highly stressed households, and had no means of reaching out. Research indicates that older immigrant seniors do not always feel comfortable accessing mainstream social and recreational opportunities. But there seemed to be an ongoing campaign to reach out to them through the hub, where they would have been made welcome.

Reports suggest that the risks of aging – both health-related and social – are likely to be compounded for Indigenous seniors who might have experienced trauma. I spoke with Mollie over lunch at a city outreach program. As a child, she had contracted tuberculosis and was taken from her reserve for two years of treatment in Edmonton. When that was over, she returned home and was placed in a residential school. I didn't hear how her life unfolded from that point. When we spoke, she had acceptable housing and was in contact with family members. But she said she was quite lonely because so many Indigenous people her age had died.

Older LGBTQ2S+ people are another group whose social lives are subject to particular challenges, often the outcome of a lifelong experience of discrimination. The front-wave boomers among them lived in a country where homosexuality was criminalized till they were in their early twenties and considered a mental illness till they were in their early thirties. The friendship networks of many were decimated by the AIDS epidemic of the 1980s. Research and media reports highlight their concerns about social isolation and a lack of support as they age.

These concerns have been poignantly revealed in focus groups that were part of one research study. Twenty-three participants, with a mean age of sixty-seven, spoke of the importance of being able to identify as LGBTQ2S+ while at the same time recognizing the risks of doing so in many social settings. They knew social support would be critical and worried about whether they'd find it. Those without children, and those who were alienated from their families, hoped for more recognition of their chosen families in institutional or medical settings.

Social isolation was a real concern, one participant said:

I often think ... is the network around me going to be strong enough and be there to support me, cause some ... many of us may end up on our own even if we're in partnerships at the moment ... and it's not always clear is there going to be a partner. We're not as connected to family as many cases, as lots of other people would be, not having, many of us, not having any children. So it's a question of is that road going to be a very lonely road, or am I going to have a very supportive network around me that helps me through that final journey.

Another commented: "We're all just human beings, and many of us have had a lot of pain and loneliness and isolation and secrecy, and it needs to stop and not everybody is aware of that yet."

I first met Rod at a meet-up group on aging, organized to discuss the experiences of older LGBTQ2S+ people. He was an activist and advocate, and in a subsequent coffee shop meeting, he had more to say. He had many stories of LGBTQ2S+ people living in isolation and fear, sometimes in "really harsh situations." He spoke of the need to bridge gaps: "Because we've been really good at putting up walls. Some of them are defence shields. But a defence shield can quickly turn into a silo." He wanted Pride-type events on an ongoing basis at the community level to allow LGBTQ2S+ people to participate – "so you can say, we're not alone."

Research on the social participation of older people living with disabilities, notably in seniors' organizations and associations, has found many examples of enforced isolation. Some were physical (like obstacles to accessibility or inadequate technical aids) while others were symbolic (in the form of stereotypes and prejudices). The research suggests that older people with disabilities embodied the worst fears of "healthy" older people.

When Russell and I met, he was sixty-six. He had been using a wheelchair for more than thirty years following a catastrophic accident. He had a partner, siblings in the same city, and two children who lived some distance away. But the problem of accessibility shaped all his contacts. "I don't visit people, because I can't get into their houses," he said. "So I don't have a lot of friends ... Isolation under normal circumstances as you get older, gets incrementally [compounded]. If you have a physical disability, compound that exponentially. So isolation becomes huge."

TO COUNTERACT ISOLATION, we need social connections. We need people in our convoys, as the social capital we can take with us to support us as we age. We need people who matter, and people who can be counted on. And as the experiences of the front-wave boomers I spoke with demonstrate, those people can be found in many places.

That's a good thing. Many of my conversations confirmed that exclusive dependence on family members – assumed to be the first port of call in any emergency – is problematic, for many reasons. Even if they are emotionally close, family members might be prevented by time constraints or distance or finances or any number of other reasons from stepping in to help.

And their stories remind us that not all social ties are the same. Friendships can develop through men's sheds or book clubs, but they might not be as strong as those with beloved family members. In Hope's case, her dear and long-term friends were in a different category from the people she knew from her drop-in choir or her aquafit class. In other words, Hope's convoy contained strong and weak ties, both of which served her in different ways. The connections we need, and how willing we are to seek them out, might depend on our personalities. How *easily* they can be found might depend on the removal of constraints and barriers like those identified by Rod and Russell.

It's important to note, too, that not everyone needs an army of social contacts. Researchers now recognize that people vary in their needs. As we age, getting rid of social ties that may be too demanding, or even harmful, can actually be healthy. Quality matters much more than quantity. But as Russell's comment makes clear, we all need someone we can depend on, or isolation will be the outcome. And some of us are at greater risk of isolation than others.

4

Thinking Ahead

Who's around for us physically and emotionally – all those strong and weak ties in our social convoys – matter at any stage of life. But they will be critical as we approach very old age. At some point, unless we die first, we'll need support – perhaps of different kinds but certainly more than most of us aging baby boomers need right now.

Many of us won't be able to manage the homes we currently live in without some help. As we become frailer, we may need more personal care. Where will we find it? To what extent are front-wave boomers confronting this question? In what social contexts are their plans, if any, being made? How are their social connections and resources shaping their thinking about the future?

IN GWEN'S CASE, A HEALTH crisis in her early sixties got her thinking seriously about life as an older person. But the health crisis wasn't the usual kind – it was a broken leg. The story of the broken leg and its consequences came up as we talked about the (very) old age that awaited us and the fact that many people were profoundly reluctant to think about it. "I think it's part of this refusal to get real," she said, "this refusal to think about their own frailties and needs down the road. It's always sort of something I think people push off, in their minds ... Especially when they're a couple. Because they have each other."

Gwen could speak from experience about the need to plan for the unforeseen. "Sometimes that happens very rapidly," she said:

> All it takes is ... I broke my leg, which is one of the reasons I think I changed my tune on that score, a little bit. I had breast cancer six years ago, and I broke my leg three years ago. And it taught me [so] much, despite the fact that I treasured always being an independent woman – I can do it all by myself, who needs any-body? – which is such a bad attitude. But those two experiences sort of made it clear to me how important it was to have friends.

The broken leg experience did it. She was on crutches and couldn't put any weight on her knee; it was winter, and she lived alone in a townhouse with stairs. She felt helpless. But her friends rallied to bring her meals and in other ways made sure she was managing. She said her thought was, "Oh, how blessed I am, to have those people in my life."

Gwen was sixty-five and recently retired when we met. She was long divorced and had two devoted sons. But only one of them lived close at hand – and there was only one of him. Friends were much better positioned to help. Though she was at the young end of the older boomer group, the health issues were "like a cold shower." She knew she would need people around her as she aged – and she had a good idea where to find them. She was looking forward to moving into one of British Columbia's newest cohousing communities.

Gwen had been part of the group involved in planning the com-munity; over years of working together, close bonds formed. She, like all the other members of the group, would own a self-contained unit. But the community was designed to be one with a shared com-mitment to mutual support. Shared space ranged from a community kitchen to places for art, music, and woodworking.

Gwen's "cold shower" experience, and the action she took as a consequence, marked her as someone not afraid to "get real" about what was coming. But not everyone thinks as she does. One of the consequences of longevity, and generally better health, is that old age seems both further off and increasingly undesirable. Very old age is in fact so often perceived as undesirable that it has spawned an industry of antiaging products and programs intended to keep it at bay. Scientists such as Harvard genetics professor David Sinclair have contributed to this thinking by developing pharmaceuticals and lifestyle regimes intended to extend longevity by keeping people not only alive but healthy and active. Sinclair's book, tellingly titled *Lifespan: Why We Age – and Why We Don't Have To*, introduces readers to "the steps that can be taken right now – and new therapies in development – that may slow, stop or reverse aging, bringing an end to aging as we know it."

Though Sinclair's background lends considerable credibility to his work, it has equally authoritative critics who challenge the effectiveness of his program. But he has a huge following all the same. In fact, I heard about Sinclair from one of his followers. When we were first in touch, Denise was seventy-four. An elite athlete in her youth, she continued her involvement in sport and participated in Sinclair's age reversal program, which involved, among other things, a keto diet, intermittent fasting, and a package of vitamins and other plant compounds.

In an early message to me, she wrote: "I'm a boomer who lives a healthy lifestyle and intend to live a looooong time. 45 forever!" Later, she told me: "I don't buy into this growing older. I think if something's wrong with you, fix it." She believed the program was working for her. Apart from helping her feel healthy and strong, she thought it was making a difference in her appearance too. "I see these people looking wrinkled and old, and I look in the mirror, and I look hot, man!"

For most front-wave baby boomers, however, Sinclair's program, even if it did work, would not take effect in time to make the kind of difference he promised – even if such an approach appealed in the first place. It certainly didn't appeal to writer and activist Barbara Ehrenreich, who published, at seventy-seven, *Natural Causes: An Epidemic of Wellness, the Certainty of Dying, and Killing Ourselves to Live Longer.* Ehrenreich, who also has a strong scientific background – a PhD in cellular immunology – writes that the book presents "the emerging scientific case for a dystopian view of the body – not as a well-ordered machine, but as a site of ongoing conflict at the cellular level, which ends, at least in all the cases we know of, in death."

This understanding caused Ehrenreich to go against the grain of her age group. Most of her educated, middle-class friends had begun "to double down on their health-related efforts at the onset of middle age, if not earlier." They participated in yoga or exercise programs, pursued medical tests, and were preoccupied with cholesterol counts, heart rates, and blood pressure. "Mostly they understood the task of aging to be self-denial, especially in the realm of diet."

Not so Ehrenreich. "I had a different reaction to aging," she wrote. "I gradually came to realize that I was *old enough to die.*" This didn't represent a fatalistic conclusion about her expiration date – she continued to eat well, exercise, and so on. But she wasn't obsessed with self-denying regimes that would only postpone the inevitable:

> Once I realized I was old enough to die, I decided that I was also old enough not to incur any more suffering, annoyance, or boredom in the pursuit of a longer life ... Ideally, the determination of when one is old enough to die should be a personal decision, based on a judgment of the likely benefits, if any, of medical care and – just as important at a certain age – how we choose to spend the time that remains to us.

Though they may not have framed it quite the same way, most of the people I spoke with would have seen her point. In 2019, a report from the Public Health Agency of Canada noted that about two-thirds of people sixty-five and older were living with diagnosed hypertension and more than one-third had osteoarthritis – chronic conditions that increased with age. (The report also noted that in 2017–18 almost half this age group reported that their health was "very good or excellent.") About half the people I spoke with reported that they were in good health. But at least seventeen were cancer survivors, and two others were being treated for cancer. Others were experiencing common chronic illnesses – heart issues and arthritis, among others. There had been at least six hip or knee replacements. All these bodies were aging.

Health issues often worked as tipping points, pushing people to think about the future regardless of whether they were ready. In an email message, Brian – at seventy-seven one of the oldest of the people I spoke with – reflected that there are two kinds of pushes. Some pushes can be put off or ignored till they became serious, such as loss of memory, hearing, or sight. (Brian's analogy was a frog in slowly heating water.) Then there are crises where the water is already boiling.

Tipping points sometimes come sooner than expected, as Sharon discovered. In her case, the shock came from a combination of health issues – macular degeneration, which seriously affected her eyesight, and a difficult-to-manage heart condition. In an email, she wrote: "My expectations of older retired life [are] very different now than eight months ago." When we finally spoke several months later, she was doing better. But at sixty-eight, she found it hard not to be resentful of her fate, when friends who had not been as careful of their health as she'd been had no issues.

Like Gwen, Sharon was long divorced, and had two children. They all lived in the same city, but both sons were preoccupied with their own lives and could not give her much support. Unlike Gwen, however, her friends seemed unwilling or unable to step in when she needed help. She thought it was because they hadn't experienced what she had been going through so weren't sensitized to her needs.

"We need to help each other, and we don't really want to," she said. "It's obvious to me now, but it wasn't before."

A few months later, in response to one of my update messages, she wrote: "I have come to terms with the fact that I am aging and that things will no longer get better physically or mentally; that my body will continue to deteriorate and I am gradually losing the ability to do what gave me pleasure in the past." She was determined to find new sources of pleasure, maybe volunteering and new recreational activities. But her experience, and her thinking about social ties, differed from Gwen's. "I am also realizing that I am alone and that I can manage on my own," she wrote. "So I am myself again. But with a more self-centred attitude. I no longer expect people to meet my needs and I know that losses will be continual now ... It doesn't seem so bad now although I do feel alone. Not isolated, just alone in this busy world of busy humans." She added:

> I have also spent the last couple of months helping two friends in very practical ways, based on my knowledge of what it is like to be helpless and isolated in a world that requires a car. They think I am amazing when I am simply connecting to people who are helpless in ways I needed help. My one hope is that others in my age cohort learn to help their friends and neighbours.

Gwen and Sharon were different people, in different circumstances, dealing with different issues. But their stories reinforced my conviction that, whether or not we recognize it, as we age, we need people, more than almost anything else we might need as we age.

ALMOST ALL THE PEOPLE I spoke with were sixty-five or older, and almost all had made the transition from work to retirement. The few who still worked (mostly on a part-time basis) were usually in business or professional jobs, where their interests were engaged and their expertise continued to be valued. This work sometimes extended to unpaid service on boards, committees, or professional associations. Two academics were writing books. Yvonne and Bonnie were both cofounders of consulting companies; they continued to be involved but both were slowly scaling back. Arshan continued to work about half-time in his accounting business. Ursula continued to teach music. Mel, at sixty-five, still lived on the family farm but was passing more of the work on to the nephew who would be taking it over. "It's something that I've been preparing, for the last four or five years," he said.

For another small group, retirement could more appropriately be called redeployment. This group included people who had transferred their skills and interests to fairly high-level work in the volunteer sector, such as the Men's Shed and environmental movements.

For the others, with working life behind them, thinking ahead usually involved decisions about housing – whether and when they might move, what kind of housing might best suit their needs, where it should be located, and so on. A 2019 federal government report on seniors' housing, drawing on UK research, suggested a combination of "push" and "pull" factors that fell into three categories: (1) lifestyle moves, perhaps to a preferred location or to enable home equity to be released; (2) planned moves, perhaps to be closer to family, or to lower upkeep and maintenance costs, or to avoid social isolation; and (3) crisis moves, perhaps due to accidents or falls, bereavement, or health conditions (including dementia).

I assumed any talk about housing involved thinking about what might be manageable for an aging body, and who might provide help when that would inevitably be needed. It might also involve thinking about existing social convoys – critical for emotional support, but not always able to give practical help. About half the people I spoke with lived in detached houses, and about 10 percent of them were the original family homes in which they had raised their children – so moving at some point might well be in the cards. Many had done some thinking ahead, though the form this thinking took differed depending on their circumstances.

Leanne, the bicoastal grandmother, focused on social connections and support as she aged, and that focus shaped her thoughts about where she wanted to live. Though her permanent home was in Saint John, and she had one daughter close at hand, she also spent substantial chunks of time visiting her second daughter and her family in Vancouver. "I'm here, and then I'm gone," she said. And that made it difficult to feel she belonged in either place. "I know that I don't have a tribe," she said. "I don't necessarily have a group that's going to notice, all of a sudden I'm gone. Because they think I'm gone because I'm gone a lot ... I don't have a regular social connection. And I know that as I'm getting older that's going to be more and more important."

To make sure there would be people around her as she aged, Leanne was exploring the possibility of cohousing – also Gwen's choice. Any form of long-term care would not be an option for her; even if it were, New Brunswick did not have enough nursing home beds to accommodate its aging population. Leanne's conclusion was stark: "Unless we become proactive and start to increase our ability to look after ourselves, and have our communities look after us, we might as well all step out in front of a train."

Melanie's thinking about the future was clear from our very first email contact. She wrote:

> I have a husband and two adult stepchildren neither of whom I expect will be looking after us should the need arise. Eight years ago we moved to [BC community] as a [pre-emptive] move. My thinking then was that it was/is walkable and has most amenities. However, I have since discovered that should one not want to live in an oversized single family home the options become quite narrow. Yes, there are some patio homes usually still too large but would solve grounds maintenance concerns but some are beyond the "walkable" zone. And also a few apartments over the shops, all being strata, non-rentals. My other observation is

I have missed the lack of diversity given most of [community] is senior.

As she saw it, the big question was whether they could "tough it out" where they were and hire help for things like gardening as needed – "and hope that I can check out on my terms and not end up in a facility."

In contrast, consummate planners such as Yvonne had moved beyond merely thinking ahead. Seventy-one and single when we spoke, she'd moved to British Columbia from Ontario six years earlier, partly to be closer to her son and his family, who lived just a drive away. It was, as she said, "a really grand adventure." But she was purposeful about how she set up her life. "I knew that being in community, and having friends, was going to be really important," she said. "So I cultivated relationships in all the different things I like to do."

What she liked to do covered a wide range of activities – memberships in community organizations, volunteering, hiking groups, music groups, and more. Because of her working life as a business coach, she also did a lot of mentoring. Yvonne's connections were richly intergenerational.

She was also in good health "for the moment" – though injuries in the past had got her used to giving up some of the things she used to do. She had no workplace pension but had some money invested, and that too shaped her future planning. She was grateful for early financial advice that set her up with insurance to cover home care. She'd put a deposit on a place in an assisted living facility where she'd have her own unit but could have meals provided. She could activate the arrangement any time.

When we spoke, she was living in a rented apartment. "Where I'm living now would not be good for aging," she said. "I'm halfway up a mountain. There's a three-kilometre walk to downtown, which I do often, but won't be able to do that forever. And I also have concerns about elderly people driving. So my thinking is I will probably be here until maybe I'm eighty, and then, we'll see, but I'll likely move there. So I've preplanned it." She knew things could change. But in the meantime, thinking ahead to that future, she continued to down-size her possessions. "And that's the other part, is that I've been get-ting used to the letting go," she said. "I think I could do quite well in a small apartment."

Critical to her planning was recognizing the need to have people around for connection and support. If she moved to the assisted living facility sooner than she needed to, she would have the oppor-tunity to develop community there too. Meanwhile, she had started a discussion group to consider what it meant to be an elder in the twenty-first century and what elders' roles should be.

For other front-wave boomers, health concerns were often the tipping point that made them consider a move. Gary, seventy-five when we first talked, had been treated for bowel cancer. It precipi-tated a move from a three-bedroom, two-level condominium, be-cause it was, in Gary's terms, not a convenient place to be sick in. Gary's wife also had health concerns. They moved to a single-level townhouse in an independent living retirement village, which also shaped their social life.

But health concerns were not the only reason people were mo-tivated to think about moving – and take action. James and his wife had also moved into a retirement community – but under different circumstances. At the time, James had still been in his fifties. The move was prompted partly by the fact that they had become empty nesters, having just delivered the younger of their two children to his final year at university. They were in the process of building a cottage and the thought of not having to do yard work in their pre-sent house was appealing. James said they "stumbled" into the move but in retrospect were glad they made it.

When we spoke, James was sixty-six, in good health, and settled in a situation that would work well for him and his wife over the long term. I thought of James and his wife as fitting into a category of people who were thinking ahead with time on their side. Sarah and Katie also fit in this category. Both lived with their partners in their family homes and both were looking ahead to retirement communities in their neighbourhoods. Sarah, at sixty-eight, could see the advantage of the family home for the present, when children and grandchildren were frequent visitors. But she also speculated about a "five-year plan" that might involve a fifty-five-plus residence in a brand-new multiage urban community close to her home.

Katie, at seventy-one, was similarly placed, in terms of family and community. She and her husband had put their names down for a fifty-five-plus residence in the neighbourhood. It had a waiting list, and she knew it could be some time before they could move, but there was no urgency.

John and his wife were also thinking ahead when they moved back to Canada from the United States in 2006. John was sixty. They sold the big old house they owned and bought a ground-floor condominium. John stressed that they wanted to stay there as long as possible. "If [one of us] was really ill ... a nurse could come by," he said. "The shopping could be easily delivered."

MOVING TO ACCOMMODATIONS better suited to our lives as old people is a complicated business. Sociologist and gerontologist David Ekerdt notes that we move through life not just with a social convoy of people but with a *material* convoy of possessions. This convoy can loom large as we approach very old age. In *Downsizing: Confronting Our Possessions in Later Life,* Ekerdt notes that our material convoys, like our social convoys, contain elements that are more important or less important, elements that are transient, elements that may have been forgotten. In later life, managing all these elements may become more challenging.

Unless we do something about them, sooner rather than later, they become a shared predicament; in most cases, family members must be called on to help. This, in turn, introduces another dilemma: possessions important to us may not be as important to those who may be destined either to inherit them or dispose of them. Ekerdt also notes that the extent of our household possessions can shape decisions about moving. In many cases, the larger the material convoy, the greater the reluctance to tame it, and the greater the likelihood of staying put – however unsuitable the housing choice might eventually become.

Take Amy's situation. In addition to intentionally cultivating her network beyond family to friends, she was thinking ahead in other ways. She and her husband still lived in the family home, which had once housed three children and two dogs. It was in a city, which in her view was not always supportive of people who were not working. She thought a smaller community, with more opportunities to get to know people, might suit them better. But the community would need to have good facilities (most notably medical ones). It would need to be near an airport, so they could easily reach their children. And it would need to be a community where they were not the only seniors in town. As to the kind of property they would like to live in, that had yet to be decided. But Amy knew she would like a patio where she could grow cherry tomatoes.

At the time Amy and I met, the option of moving was up in the air. But as a preliminary step, Amy, like Yvonne, had started the critical job of downsizing. She'd been at it systematically for about a year and a half and had reduced everything down to things she defined as "keepers." A relative who'd had to clean out her parents' home had inspired her. "She'd come over occasionally for a cup of coffee, and then kind of cry on my shoulder," Amy said. She heard about "stuff" in the house that had sat for fifty years, about a basement so full it wasn't possible to walk through it. It took her relative about eight months to clear the house out. It confirmed her resolve not to let it happen to her – or her children.

Dana had a similar experience. She'd had to clear out her father's house after his death a year earlier. The family had a long and well-documented history in the United States and Canada, so there were masses of archival records and photographs. Dana had to decide what to do with them. It persuaded her to take downsizing seriously in her own home.

Mike was seventy-four when we met. He had been treated for prostate cancer and was working to improve his fitness. His wife was seven years younger and in good health. They were living in a big two-storey house with a huge yard – in Mike's words, "like a small park." I asked about whether downsizing would ever be an option. "That's a good point," he said. Apart from the challenge of the yard work, which he conceded he'd probably not be able to manage "at some point," there was the issue of possessions. He described himself as a "hanger-on-er of things." He had boxes in his garage containing thirty-some years of work history, which his children encouraged him to tackle. We met in October, and he joked that his wife's hope for the garage during the coming winter was that it might finally be possible to put a car in it.

In a follow-up message a few months later, he wrote: "Even though I have lots of aches and pains I have not come to grips with the fact that I will be seventy-five in June and that many of my workmates have died. I just keep snow blowing, pushing snow not shovelling."

SEVERAL OF THOSE I CONSIDERED to have time on their side had people in their convoys who were letting them know what could be coming. Sarah, looking ahead to a fifty-five-plus community, worried about her eighty-year-old sister, "stuck" in a too-big house with a husband strenuously resisting a move to more manageable accommodation. Yvonne spoke of a friend who had Alzheimer's and who, having made no plans of her own, needed to be moved into care and have her affairs put in order. Yvonne and a small group of friends did what had to be done. Yvonne said it raised "big issues" for all of them, and led them all to conclude: "Wow! We'd better start taking this seriously."

Walt and his wife had bought their house three years before we met. It provided him with maintenance projects and some yard work, all of which, at sixty-six, he enjoyed. And the couple had the resources to pay for yard work or housecleaning should the need arise. But they were aware of what might be coming. Walt's mother was slipping into dementia at ninety-two, and his wife's mother had also been diagnosed with Alzheimer's. In their church group, several people had serious health issues. "We're surrounded by it," he said. "We're cognizant of what's coming because we're seeing it."

Some of the married women I spoke with, all younger than their husbands, saw signs of future aging much closer to home. Penny noticed that her husband, only two years older, seemed to be aging much faster than she was. She was concerned that he might want to stop doing some of the things they had both enjoyed (notably, travel) before she was ready.

Janet, seventy-two when we met, had been married for fifty-two years to a man who used to be a business executive. She, too, noticed her husband's more rapid aging: "What I've noticed about him, he doesn't handle stress anymore." She said:

> He's forgetting things in the house, like paying bills ... so I've had to get him to do spreadsheets, that's how I know [when bills are due.] And he doesn't read anymore. I said to him, reading is really critical ... You lose words ... Do you know how many words you ask me in a day to spell for you?

Gloria was seventy-one when we met, and extremely fit and active. But she worried about her husband, five years older, much less sociable, and with many health issues. She wondered how he would manage if she were not around to take care of things.

But I also spoke with some older husbands who were aware of the potential consequences of the age difference and whose thinking ahead took their partner's needs into account. Mike, seventy-four and recovering from some serious health issues, had a wife seven years younger. Like Penny and her husband, they had done a lot of travelling. Now, he was happy for her to do some trips on her own.

Mark's wife was also seven years younger, and both he and she had chronic health concerns. They planned to move soon into a cohousing community, a move Mark was spearheading with his wife's interests in mind. He wanted to ensure a supportive, manageable living environment for her in the event (likely, he thought) that she ended up on her own. "The important thing for me is providing a place for my wife, so she can age in place as well."

SOME PEOPLE I SPOKE with were in situations too demanding to allow for much thought about the future. Bruce, the executive director of a national nonprofit organization, was coming to terms with a recent separation, and his potential successor at work had decided against taking the job. His retirement still seemed some way off. Ian and Janice graciously agreed to speak with me even though both were living with partners dying of cancer.

When we met in November, Anna's husband was about to undergo testing for dementia. There was a form of Alzheimer's in his family, and Anna was pretty sure she was seeing it in her husband. She would not be alone in coping with it. They had three children; one lived close by and the others (with grandchildren) were in close contact. And they had many friends; Anna was active in the community association, among other connections.

But, at seventy-three, she had not expected this, particularly at a time when she was struggling to come to terms with her own later life. Her flourishing professional career in the Middle East had been cut short by war and the need to immigrate to Canada when she was fifty-seven. Too young to stop working but too old to find meaningful work in a new country, she never worked again. She found this hard to come to terms with. My sense was that the prospect of aging was making her angry and a little depressed.

FOR PEOPLE LIKE ANNA, Bruce, and others, life intervened in ways that made them rethink their plans. Plans for the future can only ever be plans; life intervenes, and plans need to change. But the ability to make plans in the first place requires a certain agency, and the resources to back them up.

Some of the people I spoke with were managing on very low incomes. Often, government pensions were their only source of support, which would have implications for their future housing options. Sole reliance on government pensions usually signalled a working past that had been low-paid, if not tenuous, and this history, in turn, could mean poorer health and other deficits. Perhaps the most extreme example was Cynthia. Her words (noted in the Introduction) are worth repeating: "I live in poverty, social isolation, with declining health, mental illness ... There's no one who will care for me." For many older people like Cynthia, the future would probably be more precarious.

As I noted earlier, there is a growing recognition among gerontologists that the word *precarity* accurately characterizes the aging process for many vulnerable groups – those living in poverty among them. (Poverty among seniors is, in fact, a story in itself, indicated by an increase in homelessness among older people. Canadian social worker Victoria Burns has noted an increase not only among those who had been unhoused for long periods but also among those who had had relatively stable employment, housing, and family relationships for much of their lives.)

A combination of financial insecurity, limited English, and social isolation has been found to make older immigrants particularly vulnerable. Precarity in other groups, such as older people with disabilities or Indigenous people with health concerns, is not difficult to imagine.

Of all the stories I heard, one of the most poignant came from Louise. It epitomized everything I had come to understand about agency, future planning, and precarity. I met Louise in 2018 at a community meeting organized to discuss the needs of seniors in our Calgary neighbourhood. In my notes about Louise's contribution to the discussion, I wrote:

> She was living in a subsidized seniors' building; she spoke of a daughter often too busy to take her shopping, and her subsequent challenges shopping on her own (she can't carry much at one time); [we also] learned that (among other financial details) she doesn't have a credit card. But she's out there, volunteering with [the neighbourhood group], and also [for social activities] in a seniors' building near where she lives.

I remembered this meeting and contacted Louise to see if she wanted to participate in my work. She agreed, and we met on two more occasions. In those subsequent conversations, I learned she was seventy-two. Eight years earlier, she had fled from a long-term, abusive relationship and found accommodation in an elders' shelter program. At sixty-five, she qualified for subsidized housing and had lived there ever since.

Louise had two daughters and several grandchildren. One daughter was disabled and lived in a nursing home. The other lived in a bedroom community just outside Calgary. She was the busy one mentioned in that earlier meeting. Louise struggled with many things, including managing multiple health concerns and challenges making friends in her building. Cliques formed, and, as she put it, "I think when you're older, it's harder sometimes to put yourself forward."

But she had one good friend who joined her on outings, and she had started a painting class, offered through a Calgary social services agency. She showed me pictures on her phone of some of her output. They were striking – not only to me but, I suspected, to her instructor as well. "I never knew I could paint," she said. It was a life-giving discovery – "at seventy-two years old!"

Though her life had been hard – *precarious* would certainly be the word to describe it – Louise decided in the end not to be a passive victim. What agency she had, she used. I thought her life was surely much better than it had been. But, sadly, more change was coming, change that would probably diminish the agency she did have.

"I'm right now having problems," she said. "I can't remember things, and I'm having trouble ... You notice how I'm hesitating over everything that I go to say, at times." Friends and family were noticing the memory lapses too. Family members had pushed her to be tested for dementia, and she'd scheduled an exam. "I'm a little worried about what's going on with me," she said. "It's a tiny bit scary. It's not going to hurt to have a test."

I recognized precarity in the stories of many of the people I spoke with. Money, health, and social relationships emerged as critical factors. But they played out in different ways. Peter had a wife and children, so he was not isolated in the conventional sense. But he was lonely and had nobody around during the day to talk to. And that was only part of the problem. Peter also suffered from very poor health; he had been a life-long smoker till a year before we spoke, and he had diabetes. Recent bypass surgery on his legs left him with pain and greatly reduced mobility. He and his wife lived in a house with a yard, and he still did the yard work. "I've got to cut the grass," he said. "You can't sit around with your feet up all the time."

It was a struggle, but hiring help, or moving, were not options. Money was a worry. Peter's long working life had been a composite of manufacturing jobs in several industries. He survived many layoffs and downsizings; the longest he was ever out of work was six months. But he ended up with accumulated workplace pensions of less than five hundred dollars a month. They still had a mortgage on their home and other debts. "A lot of people like myself get trapped into that," he said. "Because when you're working, you don't really think about it. You've got credit cards, and you've got a mortgage and stuff like that. And you've always got a paycheque coming in. When you retire ... I wasn't smart enough, shall we say, to put money aside. It was always tomorrow, tomorrow, tomorrow."

Paula, unlike Peter, wasn't lonely. She was married, and she had people around who clearly cared about her. A cleaner, paid for out of her husband's military pension, offered support well beyond the requirements of her job. Paula also had a Filipina daughter-in-law with an extended family and a grandson, who was an important part of her life. She saw her friends regularly.

But like Peter, Paula, at seventy-four, suffered from a range of serious health problems, including diabetes. When I introduced the topic of very old age, she said, "I think I'm there already. My body thinks I am." And she had so much more going on. Her son, the husband of the Filipina daughter-in-law, had died of cancer a short while earlier, and she was grieving his loss. She worried about her daughter, who was in what sounded like an abusive relationship. Her husband's health was also very poor; that, too, was a concern.

They also had little money beyond government pensions. Her fifteen-year job in the mailroom of a downtown company earned her a pension of thirty-eight dollars a month. They hoped to stay in their suburban home (made accessible with a stairlift to the basement). But they both drove old cars, and wondered how they would manage if either or both broke down irreparably. Neither would be physically able to access public transit.

Thinking about Paula's story, I found myself oddly comforted by the thought that, for all her grief and trouble, she at least had people to be with her. They couldn't solve the health or the financial problems, but they could certainly offer emotional support. Those without those emotional ties might be experiencing what gerontologists call the "most naked" form of precarity. I couldn't help seeing that form of precarity in others. Dave, with his scant family ties and lack of contact with many people, came to mind. His words, noted earlier, are worth repeating: "It's a little bit of a concern. Or a wish, I guess – not really a concern, because I've been single all my life. It's not that I really *need* anyone. [But] it would be nice sometimes too."

THE POSSIBILITY THAT SOCIAL ties might compensate for deficits in other areas seemed to be confirmed in some cases. Helen may have had no financial resources beyond her government pensions, and was renting a room in a multigenerational family home. But she was not lacking in social ties, from a beloved daughter and granddaughter to a diverse group of friends and fellow activists. She would not have seen herself as lacking agency.

Nor would Patrick. He had been a successful businessman for most of his working life. But a late-stage business failure required him to declare bankruptcy when he was seventy-two. When we met, he was seventy-five, living in a tiny, rented apartment, with no financial support beyond his government pension. But he, too, had important social ties. His children and grandchildren, to whom he was devoted, were close at hand, and then there were those dog-park friends, among others. Patrick relished the community resources available to him, even though he had no money – his local library was a revelation. In a follow-up message, he wrote:

> Life is still very good for me. Family and the dog park are my primary focus. I take full advantage of both the library and theatres to create a rich life for myself on a budget ... Because I have my health and family, mindset is what determines my reality. Due to bankruptcy, I live below the poverty line. Yet my life is rich in so many ways that I consider myself lucky and privileged.

One of the best examples I found of taking action for the future in the face of devastating current circumstances was the establishment of a Facebook group called Senior Women Living Together,

SWLT for short. Its founder, Pat Dunn, started the group in January 2019 out of despair about her personal situation. Four years earlier, her beloved husband had died suddenly, leaving her alone and financially destitute. "I was out of my mind with grief," she said. And she recognized something else: "I hate, hate, hate living alone. I absolutely abhor it." Out of those depths, she resolved to do "something that mattered, something that makes a difference in other people's lives."

Through the Facebook group, Dunn hoped to appeal to other compatible, low-income older women who might be interested in shared accommodation. When we met in May 2019, the group had six hundred members. Thanks to a CBC story and other media coverage, it continued to grow. By August, a nonprofit corporation had been created, and there were plans for a website and expansion nationally.

I heard from several women in the group who saw its potential both financially and socially. One of them, Susan, had also survived a very tough life. When I was first in touch with her, she was sixty-three. "I never thought I would be so poor, and so old!"

Susan was twice divorced and had three children. One was severely disabled, but she had raised him at home. His care had limited her ability to work. When we spoke, she was working as a nanny and living (at low rent) in an apartment owned by a member of her church. "There's no pension in staying home with a handicapped child," she said. "I want a home, and I want to be safe and secure, but it's hard to make a home when you don't have much of an income." She did not have a lot of people in her life, so she had been glad to find, through SWLT, other women in her situation. "It gives me more hope than anything else that's come along in a long time," she said.

ON THE EVE OF THE PANDEMIC, Canada's front-wave baby boomers were clearly facing a range of different futures. Some, in good health and secure in both their finances and their social relationships, seemed well placed to handle whatever might come. Others, with fewer re-sources, seemed less prepared.

In both cases, there were differences in the extent to which people were thinking ahead – or were *able* to think ahead. But the fact was that, at the end of 2019, the future was about to change. None of us could have predicted what was coming and the way it would affect people in the different circumstances I have been describing. We didn't know, then, that all our resources – but most notably our social resources – would be tested in previously unimaginable ways.

5

Pandemic Portraits

I n years to come, "Where were you when the pandemic was declared?" might become one of those historically – and personally – significant questions.

For some of the people I spoke with, "where" had considerable significance. On March 11, 2020, Nicole and her husband were in Arizona. They were snowbirds coming to the end of their time away from the Canadian winter. Walt and his wife were in England on holiday. Deepak was visiting family in India.

All heeded government injunctions to get back to Canada as soon as possible. Nicole described rushed plans and a long drive to get home before the United States–Canada border closed. Walt and his wife cancelled the end of their holiday and flew home. It took Deepak until early May, but he, too, made it home.

But for all of us, "Where were you at?" would probably be a better question. Front-wave baby boomers are not a homogeneous group, so I discovered widely different levels of preparedness. We didn't know, in March 2020, that we would be in for more than two years of lockdown at various levels as COVID-19 raged through our communities, with particularly devastating consequences for older people.

Many, like Nicole and Walt, were well prepared. They were in good health, financially secure, and had family and friends close at hand. Both, at different times, told me they felt blessed. And both, like many others similarly placed, paid their privilege forward. Nicole lived in a naturally occurring retirement community, or NORC. She volunteered for activities organized over the summer and into the fall to keep people socially engaged. Walt got his church group, his men's group, and his family organized on Zoom. Others were not so well placed. Many were in situations that were, for different reasons, precarious. Their stories of life during lockdown also needed to be heard.

The pandemic portraits that follow illustrate this diversity. I heard stories of day-to-day coping in circumstances that ranged from critical to life-upending to (merely) challenging – the kind that most of us faced. I pay attention to the social ties available to people as they made their way through the pandemic. I explore differences between couples and people living alone and the differences within each of these groups, in terms of the family and friend networks they could (or could not) draw on and the demands they had to meet. Here, precarity returns as a focus, as I consider the situation of those I thought might not be well situated to handle pandemic life or emerge from it unscathed.

Their experiences help us understand what worked for people during the pandemic, what they missed and didn't miss, and the lessons they learned in the process.

PRIVILEGE WAS PAID FORWARD when people gave support to other family members. Within family convoys, these people could be counted on. Not surprisingly, I heard many stories of parents stepping in to help adult children who were stretched, and stressed, by lockdown requirements. Providing child care for grandchildren was one way they helped.

In Ben's case, this involved a major change. His daughter in Toronto had to work from home in a demanding counselling job. At the same time, her husband had been laid off from his job and took on contract work that required him to be away from home for weeks at a time over a three-month period. For those three months, Ben and his wife stayed with their daughter during the week to care for their baby grandson. They returned home to Hamilton on the weekends.

Ben and I spoke when the arrangement was coming to an end. He thought everyone in the household benefitted and noted the close relationship he and his wife were developing with their grandson. "It's going very, very well," he said. "We are very much a part of his life now, and he is very happy with us."

For Ben and his wife, the routine meant that other things – notably, their garden at home – had to be put on hold. But he was rather sad to contemplate the time, fast approaching, when their child care days would be over. "We're home for a day, and we *miss* them!" he said. "We do miss them. And when we're not there on a continual basis ... we'll be suffering from withdrawal. We'll have to fill our time with something else."

Larry and Jennifer, whose multigenerational family was introduced earlier on, had the advantage of living in the same community as their daughter and grandson. But they, too, had to step up on short notice during the spring. Contact tracing required their daughter and son-in-law to isolate, so their fourteen-month-old grandson moved in with them for two weeks. Jennifer reported that he was used to them and adjusted quite well. But it was a busy time. In an email, Jennifer wrote: "Needless to say our lives changed exponentially having a 14-month-old 24-7."

Their daughter worked from home and had an ongoing need for child care, so after their stint as full-time caregivers, Larry and Jennifer continued to care for their grandson one or two days a week during the summer and into the fall.

Grandparents stepped up even in cases where grandchildren were not close by or could not be visited even if they were. I heard many stories of regular FaceTime and other online get-togethers with grandchildren who were acutely missed.

I also heard some charming stories of what Brian called "e-child care." Brian and his wife had a granddaughter in Germany who had to be away from school for two weeks while staying with her father, their son. They figured out a way for all three to watch Netflix movies on the grandparents' screen. They had fun choosing the movies and discussing them afterward. They spent much more time with her than they usually would. "We're having a ball," Brian said. "We would never have had this relationship with her but for COVID."

Ron and his wife also had online sessions with their six-year-old grandson. In an email message, he reported: "We visit with him without parents (working from home in the next room) weekly for 90 minutes on the web. We discuss a different country with supporting shared videos each week. We read shared e-books from the library, and a children's church bible story. He shows us all his Lego toys, and we get crazy together." Sandra reported: "I am sending my grandkids 'Gramma Math' questions every day. Then they call me back with their solutions." These grandparents recognized the needs of other family members – others who mattered to them – and stepped up to help where they could.

THIS TYPE OF PRIVILEGE paid forward happened outside of family circles, too, and through a range of volunteer activities.

Given restrictions on social contact imposed by the pandemic, and subsequent dependence on online connections through programs such as Zoom or Skype, people with technological skills were among those who stepped up. Mark had retired from a high-level job in health care administration but remained heavily involved in national and community volunteer work. At the start of the pandemic, he reported being in "air traffic controller mode." He got two of the boards he sat on switched over to videoconferencing. One of those boards later opened a temporary COVID-19 shelter for the unhoused in his BC community – an undertaking that had a "huge time impact" for Mark and other board colleagues.

Maryam got involved in a project to address loneliness and isolation among older people at her Edmonton mosque. In May 2019 she had been given the go-ahead to buy iPads for people in the group, and organized volunteers to train them. Fran's pre-COVID pursuit of a wider network of friends extended to volunteer work in her community. She worked with friends and neighbours on a project to provide snacks for the unsheltered in the local bus terminal, and actively petitioned influencers in the community to provide plans for housing them. "Thankfully, the pandemic has put this issue on the forefront of people's minds," she said.

As another participant commented, "Everyone wants to help." At a time when so much help was needed, the impulse was particularly strong. And often it benefitted the helpers as well as those being helped. This was, in fact, a major finding of a research study carried out during the pandemic by researchers in the Department of Psychology at the University of British Columbia. They surveyed more than one thousand people in Canada and the United States for seven consecutive evenings and asked them whether they had done any formal volunteering or provided or received support that day. Older participants did more of both, but age played no role in how people felt on the days when these interactions occurred – in a word, better.

Thelma – the so-called elder orphan who had recently retired and enjoyed making connections in the dog park – was a case in point. At the time we first spoke, she'd been looking for volunteer work but hadn't yet found anything she considered a good fit. When the pandemic struck, she came into her own. In April 2020, she told me, "It's as if something turned on in my brain, and I said, I can use my librarian skills here."

Thelma got involved in the "caremongering" network in Toronto, where she lived, and also in a Facebook group for people in her neighbourhood. In these groups, and also in her church community, her main role was disseminating reliable information about COVID-19 and the regulations currently in play to manage it, and putting people in touch with resources. She also posted material about the crisis of homelessness in the city – a continuing concern. "Although I have, like anybody, my own level of stress, in many ways I feel like I'm giving back," she said. "It feels so good to me to feel useful."

THE PANDEMIC'S ARRIVAL CAUGHT people in a range of different circumstances. Where they were at shaped how they experienced it. The pandemic could not be front of mind for people like Doug, whose Stage 4 colon cancer was diagnosed at the end of 2019. Treatment required at least two trips to hospital every two weeks for blood tests followed by chemotherapy, and he also had follow-up appointments. In a message in April 2020, he commented, "It has been quite a challenge to adjust as you can imagine and now with the COVID issues on top of everything else it is getting a bit much!" When I checked in again in March 2021, he was on his twenty-eighth cycle, and noted, "I have become used to it but it does tend to dominate my life somewhat!"

The start of the pandemic for Matthew was marked by open-heart surgery – a quadruple bypass. Matthew's daughter provided critical support, but the local Men's Shed also played a role in getting him through it. Members arranged for a speaker to talk to the group about open-heart surgery. Then, when he recovered sufficiently and before lockdowns came into effect, they collected him and took him to meetings. "I couldn't do anything, but it was great to get out of the house even for an hour and listen to the banter among my friends," he said.

The pandemic could hardly be front and centre for Janice, whose husband died at the end of February 2020. Her widowhood coincided almost exactly with the start of the pandemic. She commented that her grief, and the pandemic, were "all part of the same thing for me."

Of all the people I talked with, Verna's pandemic experience had to be among the most stressful and worrying. Verna was the mother of two adult children, one of whom was expecting her first baby in June 2020. Following my first check-in, in mid-March, she wrote a cheerful message anticipating some of the challenges of isolation (not hard for her, as an introvert, harder for her husband) and how they would manage the practicalities. Her son and his partner lived close by. She also had aging parents who lived in the same community, but a sister lived nearby who could share in their support.

Everything changed in April when she learned that her daughter had been diagnosed with breast cancer, which required, among other things, aggressive chemotherapy. What followed, for Verna and her husband, was a painful period of offering virtual support to their daughter (who lived three hours away) and keeping themselves isolated so they could be with her as soon as the baby was born. In May, she wrote: "I feel like we are passing time as best we can before we go to help out with the baby and see our girl. Not what I had thought these months would be."

By mid-November, the five-month-old baby boy was, according to Verna, "doing an excellent job" of keeping his parents going. "I can't imagine them going through this without him," she wrote. "I know COVID has made all of our lives smaller but cancer on top of it has really shrunk our life even more. I'm just starting to realize how much. I hope there will be time later to reconnect to a wider circle of friends."

In early March 2021, I checked in again and discovered that Verna faced new demands. Her daughter's treatments were coming to an end, so there were expectations that Verna would play a bigger role in supporting her elderly parents, who now needed much more help. Verna understood that too much involvement with the many more people in her parents' circle might endanger her place inside her daughter's bubble. She was determined not to let that happen. But balancing all the demands was very hard.

"Mostly I feel exhausted," she said. "I am slowly forming a firmer idea of what I can and can't do so that I can be there for both [my daughter] and my parents. My own mental and physical health is in there somewhere but definitely squeezed in between ... I am in the middle with vulnerable people on all sides." She added, "I'm working on giving myself some space to do nothing some days and not expect too much of myself."

FOR MOST OF US, THE PANDEMIC intruded on lives running on normal (whatever our individual "normals" might have been). One of the people I spoke with described the pandemic as "life on 'pause.'" Someone else called it "a state of suspended animation." A blunter assessment was that life had "ground to a halt."

It had certainly ground to a halt for Bill, whose major life interest was in travel and travel writing. When Bill and I first spoke, in August 2019, he was sixty-six, and lived with his wife in a small community in Newfoundland. He was planning a trip on the Trans-Mongolian Railway. He would take in Saint Petersburg, Moscow, and other places in Russia before stopping in Mongolia for a few days and ending in Beijing. This trip would have been the latest in a series of travel adventures that he described in self-published books. He also had a blog and a YouTube channel. Planning trips, doing the travel, and writing about the experience took up most of his time.

When I checked in with Bill in March, at the start of the pandemic, he had cancelled the Trans-Mongolian trip. "I didn't want to end up stuck on a train in the middle of Siberia," he said. But there was more to it than that. In an email, he wrote of feeling "really devastated" when he realized he couldn't take the trip. "I always find that I am on a real high as my next trip gets closer," he said. "This time it worked the other way. And that was before things got crazy. My travel has really defined me these past few years. Now that is gone for a long time and who knows when (if?) things will get back to normal."

In June, he considered the sort of travelling he might be able to undertake closer to home in Newfoundland. But he couldn't think about researching another overseas trip. "It hurts too much," he said. By October, he had made one local trip, done some hiking, and, at the suggestion of a librarian friend, had progressed to reading a book on travelling in Siberia. In our last conversation, in March 2021, he was not actively planning trips but was speculating about future possibilities. He thought he and his wife would do more exploring in Newfoundland. He was also learning (again) how to play the piano and, as an expatriate American, reading a lot of American history.

For other people, life on "pause" was a good descriptor. How it played out depended very much on their social circumstances before the pandemic and the extent to which those circumstances changed during the months of lockdown.

I first talked to Charlie in August 2019. He was seventy, married with two children who lived nearby, and an enthusiastic participant in his local Men's Shed. He was also a two-time cancer survivor and had ongoing health concerns. We spoke again in June 2020. Asked how he was doing, he noted that eight years earlier cancer treatment had required him to be hospitalized for three months – "so this here COVID thing is a walk in the park compared to that."

It wasn't exactly a walk in the park. His Men's Shed activities had to be curtailed, for one thing. But Charlie and his wife also had a cottage out of town, which they could visit frequently and where they could socialize with neighbours to pass the time.

They also had each other. When I checked in again, in March 2021, Charlie reported that they were doing fine. "The good news is we are still enjoying each other's company," he said. I heard more details about recent cottage trips and contact with family. "I think you can tell from my story, that we are not getting depressed and have enough variety to keep content," he said.

Couples, at the very least, were not isolated. In many cases, like that of Gary, long-lasting and strong marital relationships continued to be sustaining. In November 2020, after nearly a year of the pandemic, one husband said, "I am so thankful that I have J. in my life. It must be very challenging for those who live alone while this pandemic continues to linger. I fear I would not do so well."

But it wasn't always smooth sailing. The enforced isolation of the pandemic was a challenge for other couples who had seldom been forced to spend so much time together. When they were the only relationships available, marriages got exposed to more scrutiny and more stress. Finding ways to be alone became very important.

Anne and Donald divided their apartment so that each had their own hang-out space (one in the dining room, one in the living room). I also heard stories of negotiation and compromise, from taking walks separately and dividing up household tasks and meal preparation, to having to settle differences of opinion about pandemic restrictions. In one case, a break-up loomed – though, by the time of my latest check-in, in March 2021, it seemed to have been averted.

Couples in lockdown also had the opportunity to observe, from a perspective of love and concern, the way their partners were aging. Anna was contending with her husband's Alzheimer's disease. During the first months of the pandemic, other family members lived with them. But by March 2021, Anna was (temporarily) managing on her own, and things were going not too badly. They lived on the West Coast, spring had arrived, and her husband was a keen gardener. But the need to check up on him was constant.

The pandemic offered something of a reprieve for Ruth, the busy grandmother with an aging father. Well placed in other ways to manage the constraints, and released by the lockdown from her many caregiving obligations, Ruth finally had time to think and to spend time on her hobbies. She also had time to pay more attention to her husband, whose memory loss she mentioned in our first conversation. There was dementia in his family, and she was concerned.

In a March 2021 email, she told me that he forgot things easily and needed lots of reminders about what was happening next. "I am sure that I enable him a lot but he still helps me with my computer glitches and he's a great companion, wonderful to live with and I love him deeply," she wrote. "He needs lots of time and isn't good with sudden changes of plans. I am learning to be more patient and accommodating of him, and am happy to do so."

FOR THE MORE EXTROVERTED and sociable, however, the lockdown was hard. Even those with partners found that they alone could not fill the void that social isolation created. In pre-pandemic times, Anne had had a busy outside life, with lots of connections related to her hobbies and interests. In our first conversation, in July 2019, she told me, "I'm so social. I always have a million things on the go."

In the early days of the pandemic, she remained determinedly positive. Four of her regular groups had switched to Zoom meetings. She read a lot of inspirational material and took in advice not to focus on the things that were missing. And like many people I spoke with in those early days, she was well aware of how privileged she was, compared to others who were not so lucky.

When we spoke again in August, she drew on a quote she thought came from the Canadian classic *Anne of Green Gables:* "I am well in body, but a little rumpled up in spirit." She still had some Zoom meetings and socially distanced gatherings outdoors, so she was hanging in. But she was also thinking about what might be coming next. In March 2021, she was still hanging in but sounding perhaps a little more rumpled in spirit. "I feel blue quite often," she said. It took a meditation, or some chocolate, or some sunshine, or some time alone to get her through.

For people living alone, the challenges of social connection – and the risk of isolation – were greater than for couples. Here, too, there was a range of experience. Hope, the elder orphan with the lively intergenerational network of friends, found it difficult to adjust to a greatly reduced level of social contact. At different stages during the pandemic, when lockdown restrictions lifted, she could meet with friends. Social media, she told me, was "a black hole I refuse to go down!" But she kept in touch with friends by phone and went on a twice-weekly walk with a ninety-two-year-old friend more isolated, she said, than she was.

In a mid-year check-in, Hope told me her biggest challenge was boredom. The two things she missed most were meeting friends for coffee in the morning and spending time in the library. She also noticed something that others also remarked on – it was the social dimension of her regular yoga and exercise classes that kept her engaged. When in-person classes stopped, she wasn't interested in practising on her own. In a November 2020 email, she wrote:

> As to how life is, I would say the ongoing issue is not boredom, but lethargy. Sometimes I find I cannot make the effort to answer the phone, reply to email, or say yes to an activity. I do fight it but once in a while I give into it. If there is another lockdown, it will require some inner strength to not let one's life get very narrow.

Hope, like Anne, acutely missed in-person social interaction – what I was coming to think of as the "live" in life.

It was less of a need for others. Bruce, the executive director of a national nonprofit organization, found his working life during the pandemic challenging, but it gave him a ready-made group of people he was required to interact with. And though he lived alone, he had multigenerational family connections. He had to phone his elderly mother, instead of visiting, and he dropped off fresh food from a nearby farmer's market for his son and his family instead of stopping by to play with the grandchildren.

For Bruce, this was enough. In our first conversation, he told me he had no hobbies. But during the pandemic, with time on his hands, he started to explore a whole online world of Spanish music and culture. It was hugely enjoyable. In a message in March 2021, he wrote, "I remember saying to myself in mid-January I haven't been this happy in quite some time ... It has been a hoot and continues to be so."

FOR OTHERS LIVING ALONE, the pandemic took a different turn. Dan – the recently retired public servant who was single, gay, and an elder orphan with a small social convoy – saw himself as a "consummate introvert," and that clearly shaped the way 2020 unfolded for him.

Before the pandemic, he did some volunteering at the information desk of a local hospital and also a weekly shift at the local Humane Society. (He was a passionate cat lover.) When we first spoke in September 2019, he was looking for more volunteer activities. He made regular trips to his favourite local coffee shop and neighbourhood bar.

At the start of the pandemic, when lockdowns were introduced, his volunteer activities had to be curtailed, along with his trips to the coffee shop and bar. He had time on his hands, which he enjoyed filling by finding music to listen to, movies to watch, and e-books to read. He also spent "far too much time" watching the news. But he had no active social contacts and no reason (apart from picking up grocery orders) to leave home.

Dan was aware of the implications. When we spoke in May 2020, he said, "I think I do need to get out more. Inertia is a great force in my life." More concerning was the lack of social connection. He conceded, ruefully, "I'm not sure that anyone would really notice if I dropped dead, for a while anyway."

When we spoke again in July, he had resumed his visits to the coffee shop and bar. But later, high-level lockdowns in Ontario meant these trips again had to end. He belonged to one online group that organized movie nights and discussions, and he had signed up for an online project through the hospital where he used to volunteer.

He was also taking an online course. But he was not getting out. In an email in March 2021, he wrote: "Adjusting to isolation in the pandemic has been far too easy. Not going out comes as a breeze for an introvert such as me."

The fact that Dan did not seem unhappy about his situation is a reminder that people vary in their need for social connections. And the volunteer activities that did get him out and engaged with people – and that he enjoyed – would no doubt resume when lockdowns ended.

Gail's social isolation had been clear when we spoke before the pandemic. She had been well aware of her situation and determined to do something about it. So it was heartening to hear that this was starting to happen, even during the pandemic. Needing to stay at home was not hard for her, and she enjoyed picking up some hobbies – knitting took up a lot of time for a while. But she reported that neighbours and relatives had been getting in touch to see if she needed anything, and she was on Facebook "all the time," connecting with family and friends.

Gail's health was not great – she'd been diagnosed with high blood pressure and needed cataract surgery. But when we were last in touch, in November 2020, she had resumed her weekly volunteer shift at a charity thrift store. Even better, a friend had moved back into her neighbourhood. She wrote: "We are trying to get out of our respective houses and walk as we both need it. I'm hoping that that is the motivation that I need!"

I felt more uneasy about Dave. His social contacts during the pandemic were minimal – but they had been minimal before its onset, and I was not sure how much they would change in the future. He was one of a small group of people for whom ongoing social isolation might be a risk.

Elizabeth was another. She had recently moved apartment buildings when we were last in touch, in March 2021. She mentioned, almost in passing, that she had at one point gone two weeks during the pandemic without speaking to anyone in person.

I THOUGHT THE PANDEMIC might be a potentially serious concern for people whose circumstances I had already identified as precarious. Not much had changed for Paula. She still had serious health problems, as did her husband, and little money. She was also dealing with grief over the death of her son, and worry about her daughter's abusive relationship. But there were people around to support her. When we spoke in March 2021, friends were in frequent contact, and she had regular, hugely appreciated, home help financed by her husband's military pension. Her twelve-year-old grandson had been conscripted to do the heavy lifting when they went grocery shopping.

The pandemic was hard on Russell, a wheelchair-using paraplegic who enjoyed travelling with his wife. The cancellation of a trip to the Maritimes was a major disappointment, particularly since local travel by alternative means wouldn't work because accessible RVs or trailers were "virtually nonexistent." In a check-in email in June 2020, he wrote about taking trips into the mountains so his wife could join her hiking group while he explored the backroads with his camera. He added: "If I sound a bit down, that's part of the disability cycle. Our observation over the years has been that depression, of one sort or another, is always present as a secondary to a primary disability. It gets exacerbated when activities are choked off, the way they are now."

In Peter's case, poor health, money worries, and the loneliness of spending too much time by himself during the day were taking a toll. I noted after our check-in in October 2020:

He worries about procrastinating on many things – I think it's a sign of what many people are feeling, about one day being very much like the next day, and the next day. His daughter is still coming weekly to go shopping with her mother, so there is clearly family in touch. But I think the bottom line is that he's lonely – perhaps more lonely than he was before.

His response to my last check-in, in March 2021, also concerned me. He had new heart problems that required open-heart surgery. If it went well, there would be a two- to three-month recovery period. So he thought he would probably not return to his volunteer job at an aviation museum. "Perhaps it is time to do something else," he said.

When I first spoke with Louise, she lived in a subsidized apartment in a seniors' building. Her family wanted her tested for memory loss. By the time we talked again, in late March 2020, she had moved to an assisted living community and the testing was underway, though she was not clear on the details. In subsequent phone calls, she outlined the effects of the pandemic in her building, where lockdown restrictions became more stringent as the year unfolded. In November 2020, she was living in virtual isolation since some people in her building had, as she put it, "got sick." "We're stuck in our rooms, by ourselves," she said. Boxed meals were delivered to the door, but she didn't like what was on offer. "I just don't eat half the stuff they bring me," she said.

Family visits were also restricted, but contact with her busy daughter had always been less than she wanted. What seemed to be keeping her going was her painting. She had ordered some paint-by-numbers kits and was working on those. She told me she had her TV and music. "Sometimes I dance around, just to get some exercise," she said. I noted after this conversation that there was more confusion, and searching for words, in her talk.

We talked again in March 2021. She and her fellow residents had had their first vaccine shot and social activities in the building had resumed. She attended exercise classes in the mornings and spent time in the community room with her neighbours, where she worked on colouring pictures or doing puzzles. Meals were again being served in the dining room.

In many ways, she was much happier. But her physical health problems were ongoing. And this time, she was clear about her memory loss, reporting that her doctor had told her she did, indeed, have dementia. (Although she searched for words more often and seemed occasionally confused about my questions, she wasn't hard to talk to.) She said her daughter was about to take over her banking, and there were forms to fill out, which she thought concerned power of attorney.

REGARDLESS OF WHETHER THEIR situations were privileged or precarious, the people I spoke with coped during the pandemic. When it came right down to it, and as far as I could tell, all the coping done by the people I spoke with was successful, in that they made it through. By the time of my last conversations, in March 2021, vaccination programs across the country were well underway for our age group, and (we hoped) the worst was over.

But the coping took place in very different situations. The range between privilege and precarity was wide – and as the first pandemic year unfolded, precarity beyond anything I have noted here came to public attention. Soaring infection rates in First Nations communities and urban neighbourhoods populated mainly by low-income essential workers in overcrowded multigenerational housing highlighted social inequities and racism.

None of the people I spoke with were quite so vulnerable, and, as part of a broader cohort, their age actually worked in their favour. Most were too old to have been affected economically by the pandemic. Almost all had retired from full-time employment and were drawing on pension income. And though they had been consistently targeted as particularly vulnerable to COVID-19 infection, all but one seemed to have escaped it. In all but one case, they were not old enough, or frail enough, to be in long-term care communities.

This finding is supported by a large online survey of more than four thousand older Canadians conducted by Simon Fraser University's Gerontology Research Centre between August and October 2020. The survey found that "younger" older adults – those aged between fifty-five and sixty-four – experienced more detrimental effects from the pandemic than those over sixty-five. Some 90 percent of the sixty-five- to seventy-four-year-olds studied had experienced at least some change in daily routines, but more than 80 percent reported that their health status had not changed.

But all of those I spoke with, like older adults across the country, had to cope with the social consequences of the pandemic, and it was clear that lockdowns affected some people more than others. Social isolation played out differently depending on people's social ties and the nature of their social lives pre-pandemic.

The SFU survey approached this issue, too, by asking questions about who people would turn to for short-term help (like running errands or picking up groceries) and for long-term help, if they had an accident or a serious illness. Five percent said they would have no one to call for short-term help, and 6 percent said they would have no one to call for long-term help.

For most people, relationships and activities disrupted by the pandemic – and often acutely missed – would presumably resume, and life would go on. But it would also go on for those who had been lonely and isolated at the start of the pandemic and for whom (with a few happy exceptions, such as Gail) nothing much changed as it unfolded.

It would be short-sighted, though, to think that life might go on as before, for any of us. We front-wave baby boomers lived through a global pandemic that would now be part of our shared experience. We learned lessons from it that would make a difference to us, collectively and individually, in the future.

6

Lessons Learned

During the summer of 2020, with pandemic lockdowns in force, a seventy-three-year-old Mississauga grandmother was persuaded by her twenty-year-old granddaughter to teach Urdu to some of the young family members. The grandmother, a retired teacher who had come to Canada from Pakistan in 1971, rose to the challenge with enthusiasm. Two grandchildren lived with her, but two – including the instigator – were in Brampton, so the lessons had to be online. She gathered teaching materials, and she and the grandchildren figured out the appropriate technology for virtual lessons.

The enterprise was a great success. And it was about more than the teaching and learning of Urdu. "There was a direction to my life," the grandmother reported. "This is generational stuff. This is something they'll remember for life." The project also strengthened bonds between grandmother and granddaughters. As the twenty-year-old commented: "That's something that's happened in the pandemic for a lot of us ... We're forced to confront new dimensions of people in our lives."

As I considered what the outcomes of the pandemic might be for aging baby boomers, much about this story resonated with me. I could see (focused as I was on social ties and social convoys) several interesting shifts signalled by the Mississauga grandmother's experience: new forms of communicating emerging, existing bonds strengthening, and intergenerational connections being reshaped. Many of the people I spoke with would identify with aspects of this story and could add their own stories of change and challenge, of *lessons learned* as a result of the pandemic.

At the personal level, social learning occurred in four major areas. First, most of us (like the grandmother teaching Urdu) had to learn to communicate in new ways, sometimes with surprising consequences. Second, we became much more aware of who was (literally) around us, in our communities and neighbourhoods, and where we could find them. Third, we learned more about strong and weak ties and how, in different ways, both mattered. Here, I speculate about how the pandemic may have shaped our social convoys and our social lives in each area.

The fourth area requires a different treatment. It concerns the ageism in our lives; usually undetected or unremarked upon, it existed long before the pandemic took hold but became increasingly evident as the months passed. The lesson was learning to recognize it, not only at the personal level but also in terms of its far-reaching and harmful effects.

LEARNING TO COMMUNICATE in new ways was a preoccupation for many people during the pandemic. In one of my first check-ins, I asked people about their online connections and discovered a wide range, from avoidance to full-on multidevice familiarity. But everyone I spoke with had the potential to communicate virtually, even if only by phone.

The need to replace the usual ways of getting together prompted many people to get online – though there were also holdouts. One-on-one phone calls and texts were enough for some people. Others were game but had to start from scratch. Maryam, who worked training seniors at her mosque in the use of iPads, could attest to the need and the challenges. Some of the Men's Shed organizers I spoke with also talked of getting less tech-savvy members organized to join Zoom meetings.

Grandparents with distant and young grandchildren were among those already familiar with FaceTime, Skype, and Zoom (the three most used programs). The need to see and get to know a small, temporarily nonverbal family member was a huge impetus. So the resources and the skills were in place when the pandemic required grandparents such as Brian and his wife to step up with "e-child care."

In Brian's case, initial, intensive online care led to stronger relationships. When Brian and I spoke in March 2021, his granddaughter in Germany had returned to part-time school attendance, but he and his wife stayed in touch with her every day. They still watched movies, but their time together now also included Scrabble games and logic puzzles. "It's working really, really well," Brian said. And as he had observed earlier, it was a connection that wouldn't have been nearly as strong had it not been for the pandemic, and that initial, critical connection.

There were other long-distance connections, forged during the pandemic, that were unlikely to go away once it ended. I heard stories of contact with distant siblings being transformed from intermittent one-on-one chats when in-person visits were still possible, to regular online group gatherings via Zoom. Doug was very close to his sisters, one of whom was in England, the other in Italy. They were concerned to hear about his cancer and ordinarily would have tried to visit. They, too, discovered Zoom and had weekly family calls. In that way, the gift of the pandemic (as some apologetically explained it) was to bridge and strengthen distant ties.

Online gatherings were a small compensation on occasions where in-person gatherings would have been preferred. At the start of lockdown, in April 2020, Ben wrote to me about tutorials at his synagogue on how to conduct a Passover Seder by Zoom. "We are going to do one, and interestingly, we are able to invite relatives that are never together for a Passover Seder due to their spread across the country," he said. "We just have to contend with the time difference!"

A tragedy of the pandemic was that funerals could not be held in the usual way. But here, too, distant family and friends could be involved. Emma attended a Zoom funeral just before one of our check-ins. "It was lovely to have all those family members together when it couldn't be possible in any other way," she said.

Online improvising compensated for activities that were much more enjoyable in person. Ben belonged to a men's choir and spoke of organizing a system to allow members to video record themselves singing their parts, which were then mixed to produce a version of the choir singing in harmony. The result was "less than perfect," but it served the purpose of keeping the (aging) choir members engaged.

Other forms of online connection were forged to meet different needs. Among other causes, Helen was working online for the campaign to elect a new leader for the federal Green Party. Quentin, living alone in a seniors' apartment complex in the Okanagan and an avid novice writer, signed up for a screenwriting course through a college in Ontario.

For some, this was the period when they made Facebook their own. Perhaps because people had time on their hands, and because they were missing their usual social connections, they reached out, often with wonderful consequences. Helen reconnected with an activist friend she'd worked with when she was about sixteen, and he was twenty-one. Cynthia found an old boyfriend who lived alone and not too far away. When we last spoke, in March 2021, they were still corresponding. These, too, were relationships that wouldn't necessarily end once pandemic restrictions were lifted.

Virtual communication compensated for in-person connections but also had the potential for longer-term benefits. Learning these new ways of communication enhanced geographically distant relationships as Zoom, Skype, or FaceTime chats became institution-alized in many households.

THE PANDEMIC ALSO FORCED us to pay attention to who was close at hand – the second major area of learning. Our in-person contacts changed during pandemic health orders that dictated whom we could (and couldn't) interact with in the usual way. *Bubbles* took on a new meaning and shaped our thinking about who we could, literally, be close to.

The summer of 2020 was a reprieve for many because outdoor gatherings were possible in most places. A pandemic patio visit, or a picnic in the park, allowed for face-to-face conversations – so long as there was no hugging or food sharing involved. But as winter approached, decisions about in-person contact became more critical.

Those decisions were shaped partly by regional differences in lockdown rules and partly by individual decisions about acceptable risk. In Winnipeg, Katie and her husband had their son and daughter-in-law in their bubble and continued to provide child care for their grandsons. Apart from a couple of periods of isolation, Sarah, in Edmonton, continued to see her two daughters and their families, including three grandchildren. Mary, in Ottawa, had older grandchildren nearby but kept them socially distant at least in the early months of the pandemic.

Restrictions on in-person contact were much harder on some people than others, particularly people who lived alone (25 percent of people over sixty-five) and without family members nearby. Here, too, people improvised by expanding conventional understandings of "family" and "households." In an email check-in in November 2020, Gwen wrote:

> Four of my friends, all of whom head single-person households, have decided to form a bubble. We trust each other and have made commitments to voluntarily self-isolate, if we have

encountered a risky situation in contact with others. The rest of the time, we have each other to meet with in person, go for walks, have coffee together, etc. I am very glad to have some human contact that feels pretty safe at the moment.

Later health orders recognized this need and expanded the allowable bubble for those living alone.

Thelma joined a neighbourhood Facebook group that put people in touch with resources and help during the pandemic. Thelma's sole family contact – her nephew and his family – had recently moved out of the city. She wanted to know if she had help closer at hand. In the early days of the pandemic, when grocery shopping was much more of a concern for older people, she posted a message asking if someone could buy her some milk. In her post, she noted feeling "silly" about asking, but people responded immediately, and reassuringly. The one person who eventually delivered the milk was a young university student who, it turned out, lived in her building. "The thing about that is, I know the network is there," she said. "And I now know that there is someone in my own building, a floor down, who would get me groceries if I needed it ... if I was sick, or whatever." (It's significant, of course, that it took an online connection to set up this encounter. But Thelma noted that leaflets had also been distributed in the neighbourhood giving a contact phone number for people seeking help.)

Online postings also led to neighbourhood contacts in a predominantly immigrant community in Toronto with a preponderance of crowded high-rise apartment buildings. Concerned about the isolation and physical inactivity of many of the residents, another enterprising boomer – himself an active sixty-seven-year-old and a highly engaged community volunteer – took action. With funding from a Toronto-based foundation geared to family and community support, he made a game of getting people out to walk. According to the *Globe and Mail* story that detailed the project, participants would track their steps and report back to the group on platforms such as Facebook or WhatsApp. Weekly winners earned a fifty-dollar gift card, and monthly winners got a hundred-dollar card. The program ran for four weeks in the summer, and 118 people became active daily walkers.

Another remarkable community volunteer project was triggered by a nine-year-old girl in Mississauga, who inspired her father to help elderly neighbours with shopping during the pandemic. One thing led to another. Friends joined friends to help, a Facebook group was formed, and a year into the pandemic, according to a CBC news report, some six thousand volunteers, speaking more than thirty languages, were part of the Good Neighbour Project, delivering groceries, essential supplies, and medication to those in need of support. Chapters formed in Toronto, Ottawa, and London.

Across the country, other neighbourhoods groups organized to offer help. Some, like Thelma's group, worked mainly through Facebook, with those most likely to be isolated as a primary focus. As well as giving people a better sense of who might be around to help in a crisis, they were also hopefully laying the groundwork for more sociable neighbourhoods in the future. For older people willing to participate, as Thelma was, the potential for creating new neighbourhood relationships was there.

Some researchers express concern that all this caremongering has filled gaps that should not have been there in the first place and, more seriously, that it might not last beyond the pandemic. Some see a risk that positive media stories might romanticize the community solidarity that developed, letting governments off the hook in the future. A more positive hope, though, is that at least some of these connections will last.

For some people, neighbourhood connections were already in place. In urban areas, long-term residents of neighbourhoods like those naturally occurring retirement communities knew their neighbours, and checked in if they thought help might be needed. Those living in cohousing communities, like Bonnie, or in retirement villages, like Gary and James, knew people were around. I heard about driveway happy hours and chats on walks with neighbours – connections that might not have happened so regularly in pre-pandemic times but that would undoubtedly strengthen neighbourhood ties in the future.

ASIDE FROM CONTACT WITH family, friends, and neighbours, what most of us missed during the pandemic was a connection to people, in the collective sense. Confined to our homes, with infrequent excursions to grocery stores as our main contact with the wider world, we felt our social lives become much narrower, particularly when the spaces where we met people, either casually or for more organized get-togethers such as classes, closed or we were advised to stay clear of them. It was another reminder of our need for connection of all kinds – the third major area of learning. Hope missed coffee shops and the library, locations that in different ways addressed her need for social contact. Her recognition that it was the social component of her yoga and exercise classes that she needed, as much as the class content, was also significant. She missed the *people* in the class.

Others articulated this lack very clearly. I first spoke with Ed, a sixty-five-year-old municipal social worker, in August 2019. In my notes, I wrote that, after family and work, "the other really big thing in his life ... is music. He is in a band, goes to all kinds of workshops etc., and it's a major source of social connection." By summer 2020, he had participated in some online sessions but said they made him "even more hungry" to play live with others. In an email check-in in March 2021, he wrote: "My music has always been a way to purge my soul. It's like an emotional shower. I feel cleansed, yet something interesting is happening. I'm not playing as much as I did before the pandemic." Ed checked with a fellow musician his age and found that she, too, was doing less. "Maybe we were driven because of the gigs and jams we were sure to attend." In an email in June 2020, Penny wrote: "I was surprised at how much I missed fitness and yoga classes and how little motivated I was to do exercise on my own; it seemed to be partly missing the energy of a class and partly missing the low-level social interactions."

Researchers in many fields have picked up on observations like those of Ed and Penny. Sociologist Mark Granovetter noted that we need weak ties (exchanges of information or the extension of community networks) as much as we need the strong ties of intimate friendships and family relationships. Psychologists Gillian Sandstrom and Elizabeth Dunn build on his work by exploring the possibility that weak ties might contribute to our sense of well-being and belonging. They invite us to consider the following scenario:

> Imagine a day that begins by greeting your regular barista at the local coffee shop. You get to work and run into a colleague who you have not seen for a while, and chat about your weekend. After work, you head to yoga class where you exchange pleasantries with the girl whose hair is always a different color. Walking home afterward, you stop to chat with the guy you always see walking the pug named Wilbur. None of these people play an important role in your life, and yet a day without these kinds of interactions seems a little emptier.

The psychological experiments Sandstrom and Dunn devised to check out their assumptions involved university students, and some community members, keeping a record of all social connections, both strong and weak, over a designated period. Their conclusions, while tentative, certainly suggest that weak connections have more than passing importance, and the positive effects of weak ties may be especially beneficial to introverts. They note evidence from other studies indicating that younger people tend to underestimate the emotional benefits of interacting with people they don't know well. They call for future research to see whether older adults react similarly. While pruning social networks to get rid of social ties that may be too demanding is a potentially useful strategy as we age, Sandstrom and Dunn caution against underestimating the value of a wide circle of weak ties, for companionship in many different contexts.

Interviewed for a CTV news story at the end of 2020, Sandstrom spoke of her research in the context of the pandemic:

> I think often each individual interaction isn't anything super special ... It might just feel like small talk or a small moment of connection. But I think they add up to something bigger. It's a sense of community and trust you can build over time ... We have this human need to connect and especially right now when we're feeling so cut off, I think people are happier than usual to connect.

She thought the pandemic might be emphasizing the importance of weak-tie connections.

Communications studies professor Jeffrey Hall has come to a similar conclusion. He and a colleague also investigated the social contacts of a diverse array of people. Using the analogy of the gut microbiome (whose makeup of microscopic organisms contributes to the health of our digestive systems), they concluded that we also have a *social biome* (made up of all the social relationships and interactions that shape our daily lives) that contributes to our emotional and psychological well-being. How well-nourished we are socially depends on the nature of our interactions during the day. Those who are healthiest have contacts with close friends and family as well as the passing interactions described by Sandstrom and Dunn. They also appreciate time alone.

In an interview with the *Guardian*, in March 2021, Hall (like Sandstrom) talked about these findings in the context of the pandemic:

"It's critical to understand that we had a huge portion of our social biome straight out removed by the pandemic." Easy, quick connections disappeared, and their importance came to be appreciated as lockdowns continued. He commented: "Small talk is disparaged as being awful, but in some sense, checking in with another person and letting them know that you're glad that you're sharing a space with them is absolutely critical to a sense of community, and to our sense of social nutrition."

The pandemic deprived us of so many of these weak-tie connections – or micro-friendships, as they've also been called– that it's unlikely that we'll ever again underestimate them. Indeed, of the three main areas of learning that emerged from the pandemic, recognition of their value might be the most significant.

Beyond the sense of person-to-person connection we derive from a chat with the barista or the neighbour walking her dog, there is a broader sense of belonging that we get from being out in the world, with people. It's why we miss going to concerts, or live theatre performances, or hockey games. Penny once again summed up the feeling. She and her husband were among those who missed live performances, and movies, too. And it wasn't just the big screen, and the good sound system she missed. It was "watching with a crowd who reacts and even the smell of popcorn." The overarching lesson from the pandemic, for most of us, was about the value of social connections of every kind.

WHILE WE LEARNED TO appreciate weak ties and micro-friendships we might previously have taken for granted, closer relationships probably came in for some reassessment as well. As the Urdu-learning granddaughter noted, the pandemic forced us to confront new dimensions of the people we were close to. She learned more about her grandmother – but her grandmother probably learned more about her granddaughters too.

The grandparents who stepped up to help with child care forged stronger connections not only with their grandchildren but probably with their adult children as well. And support went both ways. People referred to adult children helping with food shopping or other errands or, if they lived at some distance, doing regular phone, text, or FaceTime check-ins to make sure all was well. Friends also helped friends.

This rethinking of relationships may have shown up the difference between who *mattered,* and who could be counted on for practical, on-the-spot support, support that all of us aging baby boomers will need if we live long enough. I wondered if adult children saw hints of their future responsibilities during their pandemic check-ins. And I wondered if people who had no people in their convoys stepping up or checking in might be pushed to make some changes.

For me, and perhaps for others, there was a final, two-sided personal lesson to be learned from the pandemic. It was about the passage of time and the need to take action soon to ensure that our experience of very old age would be different from that of our own elders, so many of whom suffered and died during the pandemic. There is, of course, a public policy side to these issues. But at the personal level, I was struck by the changes that happened in some people's lives over the time I was in touch with them. These changes had the potential to be tipping points – events or issues that might push people to take their own aging more seriously. They made me more aware of my own mortality and – the second part of the lesson – the need to act sooner rather than later to prepare for what future remained.

The differences between precarity and privilege also became more stark. Sarah's comment, early in the pandemic, resonated with me a year later. In a check-in email, she wrote:

I think at the other end of this we may have experienced a real sea change – and goodness knows some aspects of our human society need some big changes ... We (some of us lucky ones anyway) had become used to doing what we wanted, whenever we wanted, with whatever resources we used up, with relatively little thought to the consequences. The irony is that a tiny particle is bringing us down, but just maybe, doing the mammoth task of increasing our collective responsibility and consciousness.

Bruce put it even more bluntly. Acutely aware of the social inequities illuminated by the pandemic, he could see a lot of work to be done once it was over. "I think we're probably going to be out in the streets about this," he said. "If we're not, shame on us."

THE FOURTH LESSON OF the pandemic – that ageism is on the rise – also relates to how we communicate, who is around for us, and the ties that matter, among other things. But ageism's effects are so pervasive that we don't always recognize them for what they are. The headline that appeared in the *Globe and Mail* in late March 2020, shortly after the declaration of a global pandemic, probably startled many. It read: "COVID-19 Isn't the Only Thing That's Gone Viral. Ageism Has Too."

The headline topped an opinion piece by Drs. Nathan Stall and Samir Sinha, Canadian geriatricians and authoritative voices in health policy. In it, they deplored the "Boomer Remover" hashtag then circulating on social media as a comment about higher mortality rates among older adults. But they also noted with concern the widespread tendency of Canadians, in general, to see COVID-19 as an old person's illness – and therefore, perhaps, a health crisis that didn't matter too much. The implicit message, of course, was that older adults didn't matter too much either.

Older people, dismissed or sidelined, would not have been surprised by the headline. Nor would it have surprised the long line of researchers who have been registering the presence of ageism for decades. Certainly, in the decades leading up to the pandemic, there had been ageist attacks on baby boomers. Age-group stereotyping was part of broader debates about generational equity and fears that the boomers constituted a "silver tsunami" that would make heavy demands on health and other social services as we entered old(er) age. By 2019, concerns were being raised about the cost of meeting these demands – a cost, it was suggested, that would be borne by the millennials who were often our children and whose economic struggles were already well documented. These concerns got a lot of air time. A CBC radio program in October 2019 was headlined "Canada Is Unprepared for the Demographic Time-Bomb Hurtling at Us."

Some of these debates involved thoughtful appeals for policy shifts and alternative options to cope with the aging society that would soon be upon us (very much the tone of the CBC program). Others, rather less nuanced, tended to draw on generational stereotypes that placed blame for the coming financial challenges on boomers themselves. Widely circulated claims that boomers had "taken their children's future" were among the most extreme.

Scholars noted, though, that structural economic changes since the 1990s had played a role in many current inequities. Others described widespread differences within, as well as between, generational groups and noted the support, both financial and practical, that went in the other direction, from boomers to their (millennial) children. Sociologist Jennie Bristow's bluntly titled book *Stop Mugging Grandma: The "Generation Wars" and Why Boomer-Blaming Won't Solve Anything*, nicely summed up the counterarguments. But the precedent for antiboomer ageism had been established.

DEBATES IN THE EARLY pandemic months were a little different, though, because they took place during a global crisis that affected everyone. In their opinion piece, Stall and Sinha certainly drew attention to the repugnance of the "Boomer Remover" discussions on social media. But their broader concern was with the neglect of the needs of older people in general. The popular response to this neglect had, in their view, "not been pretty." They concluded their piece with a series of questions:

> When this pandemic ends and humanity survives, how will older adults view the rest of us? Will we be remembered for our callous disregard and self-interest? Or will we be recognized for supporting all Canadians through initiatives such as special hours for older and immunocompromised shoppers, or online groups of volunteers promoting acts of "caremongering?" The COVID-19 pandemic is just starting to ramp up in Canada. Right now, Canadians not only have the opportunity to flatten the curve of transmission, but also the troubling and heightened intergenerational warfare that has occurred. Let us all be more Canadian, and spread love, not COVID-19.

Stall and Sinha were not alone in their recognition of the ageism revealed by the pandemic. Other media outlets also pointed it out. And it was widely observed, and roundly condemned, across a range of scholarly outlets. Canadians were at the forefront of a group of more than twenty international researchers who published a commentary titled "Ageism and COVID-19: What Does Our Society's Response Say About Us?" Canadian gerontologist Brad Meisner noted how hashtags such as the repugnant "Boomer Remover" (along with others such as "Boomer Doomer" and "Elder Repeller") were being used "for purposes of expressing antagonistic stereotypes, prejudice, and discrimination against older adults."

The ageism was multifaceted. Public health concerns about the vulnerability of "seniors" or "the elderly" could be seen as caring and protective. But, as other critics noted, the assumption that everyone over a particular chronological age was equally susceptible to serious health consequences from COVID was also ageist (as well as being a dangerous simplification). And injunctions to care for vulnerable "seniors" could also have ageist consequences, if help (along the caremongering lines suggested by Stall and Sinha) was offered on the (unchecked) assumption that recipients were unable to help themselves. In fact, as another researcher pointed out, it was frequently older adults who were doing the helping.

This version of ageism has been labelled "compassionate." It introduces a perspective on the issue that may bring it much closer to home for many people than ageist rants on social media. The pandemic exposed many flaws in our social relationships, and the prevalence of ageism has been one of them.

Ageism shapes policies and programs (as we've now seen all too clearly in government approaches to "seniors" and long-term care). Less formally, it shapes the way other people see us. Most importantly (though we may not always recognize this), it shapes the way we see ourselves. It's ageism that makes the prospect of (very) old age so daunting. So a lot will need to change if we are to reimagine aging along non-ageist lines.

Doing Things Differently

The pandemic was a wake-up call for everyone, on many fronts. But for those approaching very old age, it was a wake-up call of a different order. Its early, devastating effects in long-term care homes in Canada was a tragedy in itself, but that tragedy also exposed long-standing, shameful deficiencies in the system. For those who might be next in line to need care, the deficiencies were particularly sobering. Along with the personal lessons we learned from the pandemic, front-wave boomers, with all Canadians, learned how many of our elders were spending their final years.

Investigations in some of the worst-affected institutions revealed overcrowding, alarming staff shortages, and neglect of residents' needs. Experts and advocates in the fields of gerontology and eldercare were not surprised by the findings since they had been sounding the alarm – on long-term care homes in particular – for years.

Pat Armstrong, one of the pre-eminent Canadian scholars in the field (and the lead on a ten-year international study of residential care), commented drily on a CBC radio program in April 2020 that "we haven't placed a high priority on providing care in nursing homes." She added: "I think, basically, we'd rather not think about them. That's certainly the case with many of my friends, who say,

'I'm never going in one of those' ... I think that we generally just try to ignore them."

The fact is that many of us likely *won't* be going into institutions that provide long-term care. According to the 2016 census, only 6.8 percent of people sixty-five and older lived in "collective dwellings" of any kind; for eighty-five-to ninety-year-olds, the proportion was about one in four. But the kind of congregate living at the forefront of public attention in the first two waves of the pandemic was only one element of a much bigger system of care, which all of us *will* need some part of at some point down the road.

The system has deficiencies in every area. Part of the problem is widely recognized. As Michael Nicin, the executive director of the National Institute on Ageing at Ryerson University has explained, Canada's universal health care system is not equipped for long-term care support. "Canada's health care system was built fifty years ago, when the average age was twenty-seven," he was reported as saying. "The average person at that time died at around the age of seventy. Today, our average age is forty-two, and we're living to our late eighties." Nicin noted that health care in those early days was approached from the perspective of a younger population, and the focus then on access to hospitals and doctors has had consequences: "We did not prepare for an older population."

One of the most articulate public advocates for reform of the system is *Globe and Mail* health reporter and columnist André Picard. In early 2021, he published a book arguing (in the words of its subtitle) for "the urgent need to improve the lives of Canada's elders in the wake of a pandemic." He, too, noted residential care as a priority when it came to fixing the system. But much more would be needed. As he observed: "Covid-19 exposed a long-standing truth: we have failed what is often called 'the greatest generation,' those who survived the Great Depression and the Second World War. And we're on track to fail their children too, the baby boomers, unless we act swiftly and decisively to fix eldercare in this country."

To repeat historian Doug Owram's analogy, the baby-boom pig is now almost at the end of the python. Just as the education system had to accommodate our numbers in our early years, so the health care system will have to adjust to our numbers as we enter very old age. What needs to change, and what options, both actual and proposed, are there for doing things differently? Most importantly, what role will social ties and social convoys play?

MANY FRONT-WAVE BOOMERS probably share the view of Pat Armstrong's friends that long-term care will not affect them. This view reminded me of a comment that Philip, then aged seventy-one, made in response to a check-in question about whether the pandemic was making people more aware of their age:

> The numbers tell me something but I seem to largely ignore [them]. I have inherited some "issues" over the years which [have] eroded my invincibility but I still go on as if it's all the same. But a little voice in the back closet of my mind does keep reminding me that I'm on the downhill slope. But for me it does feel like a slope. Not a precipice.

People such as Philip are at a critical age – they are mostly independent, in homes in the community, and probably do not yet need any support. But in the future, there will be changes. For most of us, Philip's slope analogy is a good one. If we envisage the slope as a gradual increase in the need for support, with the possible last step being twenty-four-hour long-term care, a 2018 Statistics Canada study on transitions to long-term and residential care among older Canadians offers some food for thought.

The study links the responses of people sixty years and older who participated in an earlier cycle of the Canadian Community Health Survey to their responses to the 2011 census. These sources allowed researchers to trace who had moved to a nursing home or seniors' residence and to assess what aspects of their lives might have prompted the move. Compared with those who still lived independently, those who moved were more likely to be single at the time of the earlier interview or to have lost their partner between the earlier interview and the census. They were less likely to have owned their home and more likely to have experienced poorer health or to have been diagnosed with dementia. They tended to be in the older study age groups. Immigrants were much less likely to transition to a nursing home or seniors' residence than the Canadian-born.

The youngest participants (sixty to sixty-nine in 2011) would now be front-wave boomers. In 2011, almost all still lived independently. Collectively, they were still too young to have made any big transitions. So it's interesting to consider whether, given their history as baby boomers, their onward journey might turn out to be different from what the Statistics Canada study might predict.

We can assume they will be better educated than their elders and, on average, better off financially (though there are big within-group differences). They have had the benefit of medical advances that have affected a range of conditions, including significant ones for this age group – cancer, heart problems, and arthritis. They have smoked less. Though there are debates about whether their overall health is better than that of their elders at the same age (obesity is a growing concern), they are generally living longer. Overall, according to a 2020 Statistics Canada report, those aged sixty-five to seventy-four seemed to be healthy enough to manage with little support from family and friends or from community resources.

But beyond all that, we are bringing into very old age a combination of knowledge, social connections, and background experience that distinguishes us from our elders and might, indeed, make a difference. For one thing, we grew up in an age group whose numbers and social influence gave us a sense of generational solidarity that might not have gone away. Our cohort was at the forefront of major social change during our early and middle adulthood; those of us with the resources to speak up about shortcomings in eldercare are likely to do so. (Indeed, as Bruce told me, we might be taking to the streets about it.)

Thanks to having spent our working lives in a world of rapid technological expansion, we are likely to be more comfortable with technology in general and with information and communications technology in particular. We have learned new ways to communicate that bridge distances and offer different ways to connect not only with people close to us but also with resources that will simplify daily life. To give one obvious example: many older baby boomers, in urban areas at least, are probably quite comfortable with online shopping and banking.

We also have social convoys that differ in many ways from those of our elders. We had fewer children, if we had them at all (a significant minority did not). Those of us who married were much less likely to stay married, and our more complicated marriage histories have produced more complicated families – and more complicated family relationships.

We also have diverse social ties to people outside our families. But for those of us without children or grandchildren, our social ties are more likely to be with people our own age. Because we have been aging (at least in pre-pandemic days) in a much more mobile world, our closest connections are not always near at hand.

Regardless of our personal resources, we have clear ideas about what we want. As noted earlier, a survey by the National Institute on Ageing and TELUS Health found that almost 100 percent of Canadians aged sixty-five and older planned on "supporting themselves to live safely and independently in their own home as long as possible." What we want, in the language of those involved in eldercare, is to age in place – by which we mean "in our own homes." That, in fact, is exactly what most of us are doing right now. We're

living independently in homes in the community, and we're managing it without any outside help. But we should be aware that help of
some kind will be needed, perhaps sooner rather than later. Where
will we find it?

THAT QUESTION OF WHERE we will find help leads to several other
questions about aging in place. The first concerns the nature of the
place: Is it an appropriate living space in which to grow very old?
Its appropriateness will depend partly on the actual residence and
partly on the neighbourhood or community in which it's located.
The second concerns the nature of the help: Is it the kind, and in the
amount, that can be delivered easily to people in their own homes?
Housework and meal preparation are one thing, but time-consuming
and ongoing personal and medical care might be another. And
critically, are people and resources available to provide it? Where
we age, and the help we will need, are intricately related.

When it comes to the questions about place, it's useful to start
with the big picture – the neighbourhoods and communities where
we might already be living, and where we want to stay. Here, the best
information and advice may come from urban planners and geog-
raphers, who are experts in assessing the built environments in which
we spend our daily lives.

In 2021, four such experts published a collection of research studies and vignettes about a wide range of communities. The goal of
Aging People, Aging Places is to look closely at how local environments
shape people's experience of aging. As two of the coeditors note in
the book's Introduction, "Older adults' independence, sense of dignity, and overall quality of life often manifest at the community level."
So, they conclude, "the local community becomes an ideal space for
intervention." The authors also note the inevitable question: In a
"vast, multifaceted" country such as Canada, what is "local"? Their
answer? "To us, local is the geographic representation of a person's
day-to-day life. It is their commute, their social network, their cultural

space, their familiar territory." They add: "Living in a rural community like Petit Etang, Nova Scotia, brings a different set of local opportunities and challenges than living on Queen Street West in Toronto, Ontario, or suburban Richmond, British Columbia. While there is no correct or optimal conception of local, it does influence how we live our life – especially as we age."

In 2019, nearly three-quarters of people sixty-five and older lived in urban or suburban areas and just over a quarter lived in rural areas (where, proportionately, the aging population tends to be higher.) The research studies and stories in the book explore what "local" looks like across this range of communities and in many contexts. In some of the studies, special attention is paid to groups (Indigenous, immigrant, and LGBTQ2S+, among others) often marginalized by policy-makers and planners.

Some of the challenges and recommendations are not surprising. The need for better and more accessible public transportation loomed large, based partly on the assumption that elderly car owners would at some point be unable to keep driving. Walkability in urban areas was an issue, as was accessibility, for those whose mobility was restricted. Ready access to services and community-recreation resources was also important. There were also some early signs, though, that new technology in the form of e-bikes and e-scooters might have a role in increasing the mobility of older adults in urban and suburban settings.

Housing affordability was another concern – and so was housing *suitability*. Researchers noted that some 27 percent of urban Canadians aged sixty-five and older lived in communities where the principal language was neither English nor French. When it came to housing, they were more interested in options that would allow for multigenerational living than in conventional single-family homes.

Researchers found that some communities have the potential to offer their own kinds of support for aging in place. For example, the diverse populations of urban areas might mean a wider range of services and community activities, which could be offered in closer proximity. The social benefits would include access to "third places" such as coffee shops, libraries, and parks. The researchers noted that most older adults in Quebec who lived in urban areas could access services and amenities a five-minute walk away. Rural areas, while posing challenges in terms of distance from services, had other benefits. As two of the book's community contributors put it:

> There are a few things you need to know to live well in rural Canada. These are true for all adults but [become] even more important as you age. First, you absolutely need a reliable vehicle. You need to know what to do and be prepared for emergencies such as power outages, snowstorms, ice buildup, and vehicle and machine breakdowns. Luckily, in a rural area, you can depend on your neighbours for support.

It was interesting to locate some of the people I spoke with in the settings described in the studies. Mel, who still lived on the family farm, noted the advantage of living near a paved road that led to the nearest urban centre and health care services. But the centre was an hour away. When I asked him if he foresaw a move in his future, he said, "Probably we will be moving to a larger centre just because I can't shovel snow anymore."

Amy, Nicole, and Katie all lived in what seemed to be NORCs (naturally occurring retirement communities), and the Oakridge Seniors Association, one of the book's examples, was in just such a neighbourhood in Calgary. Based on the Village-to-Village Network in the United States, the association aims to bring neighbours together in a wide range of social activities. As the Oakridge contributors write, "The ultimate intention of the association is to reconnect older people within the local area and to inspire them to become active members of the community." They add, "We are also working to develop community hubs in people's homes. The idea of this is to create an opportunity for people to meet each other within walking distance of their homes as a way of reconnecting." The potential for mutual support is clear.

Social connection, in every community, was a key research takeaway. It was found to be especially important for marginalized communities, as members of Saskatoon's LGBTQ2S+ community stressed in one of the book's studies. A lesbian participant commented: "I think that there's a comfort level for all of us [lesbian older adults] in that because we're all in the same boat and we can have conversation that makes sense with each other." A gay man commented: "The facilities that I would like to be in as a gay man aren't here ... a quiet bar or a quiet pub for gay people ... being in a crowded bar with a bunch of straight people that are 'friendly' is not the same."

Research from other sources on immigrants' experience of aging also reveals the importance of being able to socialize with peers in a culturally familiar and supportive environment. In a study of physical activity and mobility among older foreign-born adults, one participant, when asked what she liked best about her South Vancouver neighbourhood, responded: "These few blocks, these are my village. Because I know those people. [The] bus is near. And my temple is near. [When] I'm not feeling good I go there. And on Sunday I go and volunteer there ... When we bought this house, we thought the gurdwara (temple) should be near – every weekend we should go."

Overall, though, big-picture views of place – particularly the urban and suburban communities where most aging baby boomers live – reveal many shortcomings. Mark Rosenberg, a research chair in aging, health, and development at Queen's University and one of the coeditors of *Aging People, Aging Places,* puts it succinctly: "Planners and policy-makers are now playing catch up to find ways to reduce the barriers to mobility and improve accessibility for older people."

We have blueprints. Cities across Canada have officially embraced and promoted versions of the World Health Organization's Global

Age-Friendly Cities initiative, developed in 2006. The initiative identified several domains – including outdoor spaces and buildings,
transportation, and housing – where age-friendly approaches should
be considered. Social participation, respect and social inclusion,
community support, and health services were also on the list. But as
Rosenberg also notes, local governments are "not necessarily very
good at providing the everyday services that older people need." He
questions why problems such as the lack of age-friendly transportation and housing options are "enduring issues that remain unresolved
across Canada." Until they are resolved, Rosenberg concludes, older
people, both individually and collectively, might have to "create and
be responsible for their own solutions."

SOME OF THE PEOPLE I spoke with had done – or were in the process
of doing – just that. Their moves, usually from larger to smaller
residences, were a case in point. But I also heard about concerns and
inadequacies having to do with the homes themselves. Susan, for
example, lived on a low income and house-sat at low rent for a
woman in her church; she worried constantly about what else she
could find that would be affordable. Paula, with multiple health
problems, found it hard to get up and down the stairs to her basement to do laundry.

Both these problems take us to the second part of the place
question: the suitability of the home itself as a place in which to
grow very old. As Susan's situation demonstrated, affordability is a
fundamental requirement. In fact, housing affordability – classified
as costing less than 30 percent of gross annual income – is one of
three criteria for housing acceptability established by the Canadian
Mortgage and Housing Corporation. In the CMHC's terms, housing
must also be *adequate* (i.e., not in need of major repairs) and *suitable*
(i.e., with enough bedrooms for the household). According to the
2016 census, almost a quarter of seniors lived in unacceptable housing, mostly for affordability reasons, and low-income single women

were the most likely to be affected. Most were renting apartments. (As noted earlier, single apartment dwellers were among those more likely to move sooner to long-term or residential care.)

Those who owned homes that were in other ways adequate had more options. Home renovations and other adaptations could allow people to age in place much longer. This was Paula's choice. In a later check-in, she reported that a stairlift to the basement had been installed. In some cases, adaptations such as stairlifts may be all that's needed. And, indeed, stairlifts, like grab bars in bathrooms and height-adjustable cupboards, are among the most readily identifiable elements in a vast array of technological advances designed to facilitate aging in place.

A remarkable collection of these possibilities appears in a model "senior suite of the future," known as the Garden Loft, which began as a research project at the University of Calgary, led by John Brown, dean of the university's School of Architecture, Planning and Landscape, in collaboration with researchers at the university's Cumming School of Medicine. The prototype was awarded a City of Calgary Mayor's Urban Design Award in Housing Innovation in 2017.

A virtual tour reveals an array of adaptations, from grab bars, to undercabinet lighting, to whiteboard surfaces on kitchen cabinets on which memory aids and reminders can be written. A large-screen television monitor assists online interface with a health care team and provides entertainment, and a range of more sophisticated devices monitor health issues more closely.

Options such as these are at the more sophisticated (and expensive) end of a continuum that for most of us will begin with much simpler choices such as grab bars and (perhaps) stairlifts. Beyond this, however, there is a whole array of digital technologies designed to help people age in place but – like some of the devices in the Garden Loft – aimed more at monitoring than physical assistance.

Those who can afford them will also have access to so-called wearable technologies, often seen in television advertisements, that issue alerts in case of medical emergencies and falls. They form part of an expanding universe of digital supports – like a glove to stabilize hand tremors and a blind-spot detector for wheelchairs, two examples developed with the support of AGE-WELL, a network of universities and research centres dedicated to healthy aging.

In the 2020 National Institute of Aging and TELUS Health survey, more than 85 percent of respondents sixty-five and older said they were open to receiving advice on how to live safely on their own from trusted friends and family (who would, no doubt, be inclined to favour anything in the wearable technology line that might keep their elders safe). And the almost 100 percent who hoped to stay in their own homes as long as possible agreed that wearable technologies might allow them to do so. (This might indicate that most front-wave baby boomers are more comfortable with technology than their elders had been.)

The use of these technologies has limitations, though, cost being the main one. Hi-tech options are beyond the reach of low-income older people. But so, too, are grab bars and stairlifts. A report on seniors' housing needs in 2019 noted a patchwork of programs across the country, with some offering loans and tax credits rather than actual cash to eligible applicants. In general, there was little financial support to those who might need it.

THE ISSUE OF WHERE WE will find help as we age in place is equally complex. For those who live in their own homes, yard work, heavier household chores, and grocery shopping might be the first areas where help will be needed. Families and friends, if they're around, might be able to step up. But families and friends, even if they are around, might not be able, or willing, to meet all the needs that advancing age brings on.

So the next question is, Who, apart from family, might be hired to help with the range of services that come under the label of home care, from homemaking (laundry and cleaning), to personal care (assistance with bathing and toileting), to professional services (nursing and physiotherapy)?

According to André Picard, home care in the eldercare system is also deeply flawed: "Medicare may be a Canadian birthright, with accessible and affordable hospital and physician services available, but home care is another matter." He writes: "There's no guarantee adequate home care will be available, let alone funded by the public system." A 2018 policy brief from the Canadian Health Coalition noted that while roughly a quarter of seniors received some form of home care, only 6 percent received formal, publicly funded care.

That home-care services are not covered under the Canada Health Act is part of the problem. Another complication is that public funding, if it exists at all, comes from another patchwork of agreements across the provinces and territories. Picard notes that home care is the only public health service funded based on financial caps and arbitrary limits rather than medical needs:

> The practical implication is that people who want to keep a loved one at home have to top up the care provided by the state by purchasing supplementary private services ... Most home-care agencies, both not-for-profit and for-profit, provide home care both for the state and for individuals, often simultaneously. But there is also a burgeoning underground market, where desperate families turn to unlicensed care providers to save a few dollars, and to ensure there is continuity to their care.

The bottom line is that if we can't depend on our personal networks, we'll need other (paid) help instead – and a lot of it will be paid for out-of-pocket.

That's the view of Dr. Samir Sinha, a prominent Canadian geriatrician and the director of Health Policy Research for the National Institute on Ageing at Ryerson University. He's been quoted as saying that, when it comes to questions from elderly people wondering whether they should move from home (their preference) to long-term care, he has two questions: "Do you have family that can take care of you?" and "Do you have money?" His assessment? "If you're a senior in this country, those are the two elements that will determine your future."

Certain groups are seriously affected by this reality. According to the 2018 policy brief noted above, low-income, racialized, Indigenous, and LGBTQ2S+ seniors have greater problems accessing quality care, and single and immigrant seniors are particularly vulnerable to financial stress.

At least until the pandemic struck, the big question about home care was who was providing it. A significant proportion of paid care workers – called personal support workers (PSWs) or care aides, among other terms – were racialized women struggling to survive on inadequate wages in part-time jobs. Many juggled multiple jobs both in private homes and long-term care institutions to cobble together a wage they could live on. "Personal care workers are ubiquitous in the health system: in long-term care homes, home care, correctional facilities, hospitals and more," writes Picard: "These hard-working women are paid lowly wages for back-breaking work, and are largely taken for granted both by the individuals they serve and by the institutions that employ them, as well as by a society whose policies and values have made this work a cornerstone of eldercare."

Already in short supply for home-care clients, by mid-2021 their numbers seemed likely to drop even more. In Ontario, for example, PSWs could earn an average of five dollars an hour more in long-term care homes than in community settings because the province, dealing with a long-term care system (and staffing levels) devastated by the pandemic, set up financial and educational incentives to recruit them. Sue VanderBent, the CEO of Home Care Ontario, expressed concern about the effects on the home-care system. "We've got to work really hard to recruit and retain and repatriate because a lot of people have left home care," she said. "This wage differential will cause a cascade."

It's not hard to see why. In another media interview, Connie Ndlovu, who worked as a PSW in the Toronto area, put it bluntly: "Most people working in home care are predominantly women of colour and they are forgotten. The wages are crappy wages, the working conditions are exploitive and the funding doesn't sustain any benefits for these women." No wonder they were moving.

WITH PAID HOME CARE inadequately supported and staffed, it's no surprise that family members have been carrying a heavy caregiving load. As noted earlier, only 6 percent of the roughly one-quarter of seniors receiving home care in 2016 got it from paid workers. Care for the rest, according to the Canadian Health Coalition policy brief, came "informally through family or friends, most of whom are women."

The numbers tell some of the story. In 2018, according to a Statistics Canada survey, almost one in four Canadians aged fifteen and older were providing care to a family member or friend with a long-term health condition, a physical or mental disability, or problems related to aging. Almost half (the majority of them between the ages of forty-five and sixty-four) were caring primarily for their parents or parents-in-law. They typically spent four hours a week on caregiving responsibilities. For this category of caregivers, the most common type of help (reported by 84 percent) was transportation (errands, shopping, or attending medical appointments); 64 percent reported helping with meal preparation and house cleaning.

According to the report, about 70 percent of caregivers said they received some kind of support or assistance for their caregiving duties – often from a spouse or partner, their children, or other family members. But about one-third reported that they didn't get as much help as they needed. What was lacking, in 68 percent of cases, was financial support, government assistance, or tax credits; for 40 percent, it was home care; for 39 percent, it was information and advice; and for 36 percent, it was help from medical professionals.

The numbers tell some of the story. But what's most significant, now, is the story that the numbers don't tell. For one thing, they don't expose the public policy push to encourage family caregivers to assume responsibility and pick up the slack. This push is neatly exemplified on a "Caregiver Readiness" link on the Canada Employment and Social Development website. The page includes a video on "How to Be the Best Caregiver Possible: Tips and Tricks."

The numbers also don't relate to the age group – front-wave baby boomers – who will need care in the future and who are differently situated in terms of family support. There's now growing awareness, among researchers at least, of the demographic characteristics of the baby-boom cohort – fewer family ties, adult children's geographic mobility and increased labour force participation, more complicated family relationships – that may make family members much less available to be caregivers in the future. As one study put it: "One might conclude that while the policy context is one of 'family care by stealth,' the demographic context is of 'stealthily disappearing family carers.'"

So Connidis's discussion of who counts as family bears revisiting. In the present demographic context, Connidis argues that it will be important to be as inclusive as possible:

> Rather than assume that only those who are married or in legally recognized relationships have a partner, counting those who cohabit and LAT [live apart together] as well as marry reveals who really has a partner and who does not. Siblings can also be important peers for those who do not have a partner. Rather than focus on counts of children as though they are the only ties with a younger generation, we must also count other intergenerational kin, including step ties, children-in-law, nieces and nephews, and grandchildren. Recognizing the negotiated family ties of

those who have been excluded historically, such as those who are LGBTQ, also provides important baseline information about family networks.

But Connidis and others also note that there are many questions that need to be answered. Will the apparently extended family networks created by multiple marriages and step-relationships mean more people available to provide care? Or will the presence of extra sets of older people in adult children's convoys mean less time available and, inevitably, more stress on their own families? How will caregivers balance caregiving responsibilities with workplace demands? How will sibling relationships bear up when there are fewer of them to share care? And in the absence of family networks, even of the most inclusive kind, what role might older people's friendship networks play? Finally, and critically, what about those who have nobody to turn to?

With these questions in mind, a finding from the National Institute on Ageing and TELUS Health survey is thought-provoking: only 31 percent of Quebec respondents and 47 percent of respondents in the rest of Canada said they were personally and financially prepared to become a caregiver for an aging family member. Those not prepared may well be loving and caring adult children who simply can't take on the work. This is the point when older people's social ties and social convoys take on new significance.

I thought of all the people I'd spoken with and tried to imagine what support might be available to them. They represented the full gamut of connections. Jennifer and Larry were secure in a multigenerational family and had adult children who had already announced their intention of caring for them as they aged. Anna, who lived with a husband with dementia, had three devoted daughters, including one close at hand. Matthieu, in a long-term gay relationship, had no children but a close extended family of siblings, nieces, and nephews. Melanie had two stepchildren but didn't expect either of them to provide care for her or her husband if the need arose. Hope, the elder orphan, had no family ties but a wide multigenerational group of close friends.

Others, with few if any close ties, were in much more precarious situations. And it wasn't just a matter of having nobody to take on some caregiving. It was having nobody available to advocate on their behalf. Leslie, who lived alone in poor health and with no money, described this as one of her biggest fears.

FOR FRONT-WAVE BABY boomers, the prospects for aging in place could be fraught with challenges. Communities have been slow to adopt age-friendly practices, and individual homes often present problems too. Affordable housing is in very short supply. Add in the inadequacies in home care and the potentially diminishing availability of family members and friends, and the picture does not look bright.

Indeed, all these deficiencies were often what sent older people into long-term care institutions in the first place. The Canadian Institute for Health Information estimated in 2020 that one in nine newly admitted long-term care residents could potentially have been cared for at home. Picard's sources put the proportion much higher.

That fact, along with the devastation in long-term care homes wrought by the pandemic, has produced a change in thinking about how eldercare should be delivered – a change that, with enough political will and a lot of luck, might make a big difference to the experience of us front-wave baby boomers entering very old age. Long-term care homes, as noted earlier, will be getting priority attention. But there's also growing recognition of the changes needed, at several levels, to enable the aging in place that we would prefer.

Some of those changes will need to address community- and residence-related issues. In his book, Picard offers a succinct summary that starts right at home. He calls for modified building codes "so that features such as doorways wide enough for wheelchairs, ramps, and grab bars in tubs and showers become standard features instead of ones that require costly renovations." He has other suggestions at the municipal level:

> Municipalities, if they value seniors, need to prioritize services like sidewalk clearing, well-lit streets and public transport. Inclusivity needs to be built in to public policies. Being senior-friendly also means bringing services to people instead of making them travel. The main reason elders are driven out of their homes is not illness but everyday barriers to getting round in the community, such as insufficient public transportation and the lack of enough restrooms and elevators in public spaces.

In all these areas, there are models for change and pressure in the right circles to keep change coming. Much of the change at the municipal level focuses on the principles of universal design – in short, design that makes buildings and communities accessible to everyone, no matter the physical limitations they may have.

Beyond design issues, aging in place in any sort of housing, according to a group of researchers at Queen's University, rests on people having a sense of autonomy and independence, so they can be actively involved in making decisions about themselves and their communities. They also need to be able to build supportive social networks. The researchers describe two existing models of communities along these lines. The first, founded in the United States, is the village model (on which the Oakridge community in Calgary was based). "Villages" develop in neighbourhoods of single-unit homes and involve older adults getting together as a group to organize paid and volunteer services. The other model, founded in Denmark, and now flourishing in Canada, is the cohousing community.

When I spoke with Bonnie, she lived in a cohousing community in British Columbia (where the movement is particularly strong). Gwen and several other people I spoke with were also prospective cohousing residents. They chose these communities precisely because they were *communities,* offering independent living in a context of mutual sharing and support.

The researchers also identify naturally occurring retirement communities, or NORCs, as offering "enormous" potential if neighbours choose to come together to support one another. Amy, Nicole, and Karen lived in suburban communities of single-family homes where neighbours knew neighbours and were prepared to know them better as they all aged in place.

But the researchers describe another kind of NORC, created a decade ago by the older residents of a Kingston apartment building. Together with a community board of directors and an onsite coordinator, the residents ran community activities, including physical and social activities and congregate dining, in a common space donated by the building's landlord. Through collaboration with the Queen's researchers, and others from McMaster University and Western University, by 2020 their model had been extended to six new NORCs in Ontario.

But for many older people on low incomes, aging in place will only be possible if housing is affordable. Picard notes that the City of Toronto, with a population of 3 million people, had only eighty-three buildings with subsidized spots for seniors. These buildings housed some 12,500 elders – but nearly 11,000 more were waiting for a place, and there was a ten-year wait list. For those on the list, moving in with family members or finding a place in an institution might be the only options.

AGING IN PLACE WILL ALSO BE possible only if deficiencies in home care are addressed. Thanks to the pandemic, the advantages of supporting older people in their homes have become clear, and the options are straightforward. Personal support workers, or PSWs, at the heart of home-care delivery, need more support. As Pat Armstrong observed in her CBC interview, personal care work is skilled work – "whether it's the skill in cleaning, or serving food, or in providing bed care." Lifting a body, she added "is not the same as lifting a sack of potatoes. Persuading someone to let you bathe them is a skilled job." PSWs' skills need to be rewarded appropriately, with full-time jobs and adequate incomes, job security, and benefits. These strategies might also attract more workers – and more workers will be needed as front-wave baby boomers enter very old age.

Support also needs to be given to family caregivers, whose challenges are now well known. The 2020 National Seniors' Strategy developed by the National Institute on Ageing reinforces the point, noted earlier, that most care provided to older people in Canada comes from family and friends – care worth about $9 billion in 2019. At least 6 million working Canadians are estimated to be juggling unpaid caregiving with their employment duties.

The strategy document notes that caregivers' continuing dedication provides a greater level of care but takes "an enormous toll" on their personal health, well-being, and finances. The document includes a wide range of recommendations for support in the form of workplace programs for those still working, and more formal recognition, standards, and financial support at the federal and provincial or territorial level.

The strategy document also notes that while the number of older Canadians requiring the support of unpaid caregivers is projected to more than double by 2050, recent estimates suggest there will be 30 percent fewer close family members – notably, spouses and adult children – available to provide care. Increasingly, the care work currently provided by family caregivers will need to be supplemented by paid care workers. And even in the shorter term, front-wave baby boomers without adult children, or without family members close at hand, will need care-worker support.

The need to weave all the aspects of caring at home into an integrated system is clearly articulated by Ai-Jen Poo, an American labour activist whose work with US domestic workers led to the formation of the National Domestic Workers' Alliance. She is also the codirector of Caring Across Generations, a coalition of advocacy organizations working to transform the long-term care system in the United States. Its focus is on the needs of aging Americans – but much of what she has to say applies in Canada.

In her book *The Age of Dignity*, she calls for a "care grid," which would bring together public, private, and nonprofit resources into a "comprehensive, co-ordinated system in which elders can age with dignity and their caregivers, both professional paid workers and unpaid family or friends, can thrive as well." The main goals of the care grid are clear:

> We know we need more jobs in home care. We know we need home care to be affordable, easily accessible, and delivered at the highest quality. We need these jobs to be well-respected and secure with living wages, benefits, security, and opportunities for job advancement. We need the workforce to be prepared, trained, and adaptive to the particular needs of the individuals and families they are supporting. And we need for everyone to feel like whole and equal parts of a care team.

The financial support needed to bring home care to this level would be considerable – but these costs need to be compared to the cost of long-term care, which would be the only option for many seniors otherwise. Canada currently spends one dollar on home care for every six dollars spent on long-term care – a ratio that puts us at odds with most other developed countries. Don Drummond and Duncan Sinclair – research experts in, respectively, global public policy and health services and policy at Queen's University – note that the countries most highly regarded for their eldercare (for example, Denmark and the Netherlands) do the reverse; they spend far more on home care than on long-term care. Canada, they argue, should do the same. With the number of baby boomers heading into very old age, the "warehousing" practices of the past just aren't feasible or affordable: "The cost of institutional accommodation and care – to residents, their families and the public purse – exceeds by far what it would cost to provide an extended range of seniors' needs through beefed-up home and community support services. That would be expensive too, but it's an approach to helping our seniors age well that our country could afford."

There are signs that we may be moving in the direction the experts recommend. The federal government's 2021 budget began with an apology to seniors, especially those in long-term care, by finance minister Chrystia Freeland. It promised $3 billion in additional funding to improve the quality and infrastructure of long-term care systems, and $90 million over three years to support older Canadians (particularly those on low incomes) to age at home. This would be a very good start.

PHILIP'S COMMENT ABOUT THE "slope" of change may well apply to many of us front-wave baby boomers. But with enough political will and good luck (and, if necessary, the taking-to-the-streets advocacy of boomers themselves), our "fourth age" might look different from the version, exposed by the pandemic, that is the only option for many of our elders.

It's worth repeating that in 2016 only about 7 percent of those sixty-five and older, and about 25 percent of those aged eighty-five to ninety, were living in congregate settings. In years to come, there will be many more of us in those older age groups. More of us will need home care than long-term care. But some of us *will* need long-term care, if our health fails or (probably the most frightening prospect for most of us) if we develop dementia. So it's comforting to think that the institutional silos at the forefront of our attention during 2020 may not be around, at least in the same format. As Picard puts it: "After decades of duct tape solutions, Canada's provinces need to make judicious use of the wrecking ball. What needs to replace many of our large, decrepit institutions are smaller, more homelike facilities that are built to the needs of residents."

In any upgrading, Picard has a list of elements that should become standard. They include "private or semi-private rooms and bathrooms, homey communal spaces, ready access to the outdoors, air conditioning, non-slip floors, laundry and cleaning services, and in house foods." And there is another critical requirement: "Nursing homes should be an integral part of the community, not hidden away."

The call for smaller, community-based care facilities is widespread, and there are many models. Pat Armstrong and her colleagues have concluded a ten-year international study of residential care and developed a collection of promising practices from observations and field work in Canada, the United States, the United Kingdom, Germany, Sweden, and Norway. The aim of the study, in the words of research team member Donna Baines, was to "build a vision of what high quality care could look like." The promising practices had to meet three principles: they had to treat both residents and providers with dignity and respect; they had to understand care as a relationship; and they had to take differences and equity into account.

The promising practices cover a wide range. In a small town in Norway, a twenty-four-bed nursing home has been fully integrated into a community centre that includes a day care centre and swimming pool; across the square, residents have access to a cinema, bookstore, hairdresser, and other businesses. Armstrong noted: "The physical integration with the community was particularly impressive, providing an excellent model for bringing generations as well as activities together."

In a nursing home in a big city in Sweden, good staffing levels make it possible for workers to spend time on caring. Each nine-resident unit has one resident nurse in charge and three assistant nurses who work during the day. The home had also introduced a new staffing schedule to ensure that residents see the same staff as much as possible.

There are also promising practices in Canadian care homes. In one BC nonprofit long-term care home, careful attention is paid to diet and nutrition. Food comes from local sources, including some grown by residents themselves in the home's garden. Staff developed an "Asian Fusion" cuisine for the more than 50 percent of residents of Asian origin.

At a personal care home in Manitoba, all staff – from management to laundry and housekeeping – are employees of the organization, and all are encouraged to have daily contact with residents. The division of labour is blurred: registered nurses and licensed practical nurses work together on practical and administrative chores. Staff turnover is low.

What the researchers found to be critical to the success of any residence – on top of considerations such as the physical environment or the attention to food and laundry – is the availability of enough staff to spend time with residents and develop relationships with them. It makes all the difference.

TORONTO STAR JOURNALIST Moira Welsh can also attest to the existence of models, in Canada and elsewhere, for doing long-term care differently. After writing about nursing homes in Ontario for nearly two decades, she noted that her stories "always exposed the negative." Then came the pandemic and its disastrous consequences for people in long-term residential care. Persuaded that bad news stories would not bring about change, and persuaded too of the need to put stories of positive change into the public domain, she set out to find places where positive change might be happening, and the people who were working to bring it about. The result was a book, published in 2021, called *Happily Ever Older: Revolutionary Approaches to Long-Term Care*. It contains inspiring examples, from the United States, Europe, and Canada, of long-term care arrangements that are homelike and built on the sort of caring relationships Armstrong and her team strongly advocate.

In Canada, for example, several Ontario nursing homes have adopted an approach to care for people with dementia based on a UK model calling for homelike, rather than hospital-like, environments and relationships. It transformed the way staff – all staff – interact with residents.

Another Canadian example, now gaining international prominence as a model, is the Sherbrooke Community Centre in Saskatoon. Residents, many with dementia or mild cognitive decline, live in little homes, each with its own kitchen, a family room, and a door to an outdoor garden. Workers cook meals to residents' tastes, and in the process of caring for them, come to know them as people, as interesting and valued in very old age as they ever were when they were younger. Sherbrooke's approach is built on a philosophy of caring, well known in the United States and increasingly in Canada, too, as the Eden Alternative. It represents a huge shift away from the hospital-style institutional settings that have dominated long-term residential care in Canada. It is an inspiring model.

But it is only a model. Welsh notes that much of the work to bring about change, based on models like the Eden Alternative, is being done by a handful of passionate advocates, often in their own programs. Funding in many cases is a challenge. While the need for change is now widely recognized, the means to bring it about on a scale that will soon be needed in Canada remains an enormous challenge. In the epilogue to her book, Welsh writes: "Let's be blunt. If the boomers and those who will follow want to change the way they live in their elder years, we'd all better start agitating for change right away. It takes time to enact real change, and we don't want to get to our older, frailer, quieter stage without those improvements in place."

8

Reimagining Aging

began work on this book in early 2019, with the goal of exploring what (very) old age might be like for the huge cohort of front-wave baby boomers about to enter that stage. It's interesting now to speculate on what I might have discovered had a global pandemic not upended the project and raised many sobering questions in the process.

That initial goal still led to some important discoveries. My conversations with a wide range of boomers across the country illustrated how diverse the cohort was. The group conventionally described as "seniors" or "the elderly" were far from homogeneous. Their differences, across a wide range of characteristics, made it clear that their needs as they aged would differ too. The privilege and precarity that emerged in many stories would uncover big differences in the way individuals experienced aging. Their sheer numbers would pose problems of scale not previously encountered in the world of eldercare. And they would be growing old in family and social circumstances that hinted at much less informal support.

But as a result of the pandemic, the *context* in which people might imagine growing old also began to change. In fact, everything to do with aging seemed to come into question. Aging, in effect, was being reimagined.

Much of that reimagining involved a commitment to finding new ways to organize eldercare. But another side of the issue, seldom addressed, relates to the pervasive ageism that shapes how we think about old people – and how we think about ourselves. The recognition of ageism is one of the lessons we learned from the pandemic. Here, I look at the reimagining that must happen to do away with ageism – and change the way aging is experienced for everyone.

IN MARCH 2021, A COLUMN appeared in the *Toronto Star* about the potential challenges of registering for Ontario's vaccine rollout. Columnist Emma Teitel wrote: "It appears that in the absence of a streamlined, universal vaccine registration process from the get-go – one that our parents may have had an easier time accessing – there is us: millennials frantically signing our boomer parents up for shots. I bet you 100 shares of Pfizer Inc., that behind every vaccinated 70-year-old is a 30-year-old on an iPhone."

Teitel would have lost her bet. A few days later, the newspaper published a terse response from a seventy-eight-year-old who found the provincial website easy to use: "I'm tired of the casual ageism in our society that makes it so easy for Emma Teitel to write: 'I bet you ... that behind every vaccinated 70-year-old is a 30-year-old on an iPhone.' Does she think that everyone who used a computer for their jobs suddenly loses this skill when they turn 70?"

Where does this kind of thinking come from? Psychologically, we have a tendency, nicely illustrated in the Teitel column, to segregate people into age groups and then to make judgments about the group as a whole. Our judgments are stereotypes, but they're not straightforwardly positive or negative. Instead, researchers have found they tend to be a nuanced mix of perceptions along two dimensions: warmth and competence. When it comes to aging, older people tend to be seen as warm or likeable but incompetent or dependent. Clearly, that's not always the case. So those offers of help, however well-intentioned, may be patronizing and may ultimately do more harm than good.

But stereotypes along these lines are only part of the story. *Ageism* as a term is generally acknowledged to have been coined in 1968, by US medical doctor Robert Butler. He was expressing his concern about reactions (from middle-class, middle-aged white residents) to a plan for subsidized housing for older people in an affluent neighbourhood near Washington, D.C., and used the term to explain what he thought was going on.

Butler went on to have a long career in aging research and geriatrics and contested ageism wherever he saw it. In 1989, he defined ageism more formally as "a systematic stereotyping of and discrimination against people because they are old, just as racism and sexism accomplish this with skin colour and gender." Ageism, for Butler, showed itself in "a wide range of phenomena, on both individual and institutional levels – stereotypes and myths, outright disdain and dislike, simple subtle avoidance of contact, and discriminatory practices in housing, employment and services of all kinds." He thought that it might parallel racism as "the great issue of the next 20 to 30 years."

In his original 1969 article, he was even more direct about its implications. Ageism, he wrote, reflected "a deep seated uneasiness on the part of the young and middle-aged – a personal revulsion to and distaste for growing old, disease, disability; and fear of powerlessness, 'uselessness,' and death." The sad irony is that it isn't only the young and the middle-aged who express this distaste. Extended longevity has led to a denial of the "fourth age" on the part of many of us front-wave baby boomers, for all the reasons Butler outlined.

In the Introduction to this book, I quote US antiageism writer and activist Ashton Applewhite, whose book *This Chair Rocks: A Manifesto against Ageism* (2016) articulates many arguments worth making here. She writes:

Unless we confront these expectations of impairment and in-
significance, they build up over the decades, making older adults
themselves the worst ageists of all. We rule out activities or outfits
or relationships preemptively because they might not be "age-
appropriate," especially with any tinge of sexuality – a double
taboo. Over time, as age-related stereotypes grow more relevant,
people tend to act as though they were accurate, creating self-
fulfilling prophecies.

Applewhite's advice to older people is to push back against the stereotypes, to reject the "bogus" young-old binary, and to be open to
the positive side of getting older. In her words: "The sooner growing
older is stripped of reflexive dread, the better equipped we are to
benefit from the countless ways in which it can enrich us."

ONE OBVIOUS STRATEGY to help end ageism for everyone is to end
the age segregation that produces those stereotypes in the first place.
This can happen at many levels, starting with the big picture – where
people live. We saw the separation and isolation of older adults living in long-term care homes and other congregate settings during
the pandemic. That has inspired widespread calls for change. André
Picard argues: "We need to stop with the elder apartheid and inte-
grate care homes into the community." He suggests that facilities
should be shared with daycares and schools.

Care homes are a place to start. But most older people live in the
community – a trend that we front-wave boomers intend to continue. We want those communities to be age-friendly – and that has
the potential to make them less age-segregated too. As Applewhite
also points out, "Age-friendly communities aren't just wheelchair- and
walker-friendly, they're gurney- and skateboard- and stroller- and
bus passenger- and delivery-guy- and tired-person-friendly. Let's call
these programs what they are – *all*-age-friendly."

Beyond physical and structural changes, there are many ways of bringing generations together close to home – and ditching stereotypes in the process. Among the people I spoke with, there were examples of multigenerational family living – more common in Indigenous and immigrant communities but perhaps likely to become more widespread as a result of the pandemic. It's a trend *Globe and Mail* columnist Elizabeth Renzetti strongly endorses in an opinion piece describing her own extended family's experience. While noting the persistence of an "odd North American aversion" to multigenerational living, she writes: "I'm here to tell you why that is a pile of hooey, and why you should defy the cold individualism of the day and bring your family members closer."

But families don't have a monopoly on multigenerational living. Several of the people I spoke to lived in multigenerational settings with people who weren't family. Helen rented a room with a family. Bonnie lived in a cohousing community where residents ranged in age from teenagers to people in their eighties. Narek rented rooms to young tenants, one of whom had just aged out of foster care.

A CBC program in April 2021 described a couple who "adopted" their widowed, childless friend, then in her late sixties, and took her to live with them when they moved provinces. The arrangement had lasted twenty years. One of the partners commented: "This is the elder that I love, who is first in my heart, who I will commit myself to seeing to the end of her days." The other thought their story showed an alternative to eldercare and said it "beats putting them in the old age home." She called for more help from all levels of government to make this option more feasible for more interested Canadians. "Maybe it takes a village also to keep an elder, not just to raise a child," she said.

But, of course, intergenerational housing isn't the only way age segregation can be upended. It's here that intergenerational relationships are so important. And they need to be *relationships,* even of the weak-tie variety, not fleeting encounters or connections borne of compassionate ageism. I talked to people with and without young family members who were actively engaged with younger people – none of whom were likely to see them as frail or impaired or, indeed, as anything but *who they were*. Diana was seventy-three when she showed me the video of her young international student tenants dancing with her in her kitchen. Ursula, at sixty-eight, had ongoing connections to present and former music students. Paul, at seventy-one, was a busy volunteer grandparent. And there were many others.

Establishing those intergenerational connections takes work. For those without young family members, the tendency is to associate with people of the same age; those are the connections that may be easiest and most comfortable. The phenomenon of age homophily captures this tendency. Research in the area has found that shared interests are a good way to cross age barriers and develop intergenerational connections – a finding also reinforced by some of the people I spoke with.

Hope was a strong advocate for intergenerational ties. She found many of hers when she volunteered on an urban farm in her late sixties. It meant working constantly with young people who were "true believers," set to change the world. The fact that Hope shared their interest links to the broader point, established by many researchers, that wanting to change the world is something many older adults share with younger ones. Though a tendency has been noted among some young climate activists to take on the "OK Boomer"/intergenerational unfairness perspective and blame "older people" for being indifferent to climate change, in fact, young activists have many older supporters. A charming video conversation between climate change activist Greta Thunberg and veteran UK natural historian and broadcaster David Attenborough makes this point.

Joint work on environmental or other political campaigns, joint community development initiatives (such as a BC Men's Shed supporting Syrian refugee families), even those dog park conversations that bring all ages together are among the many ways people are finding intergenerational connections. If there were enough of them, ageism would be very hard to sustain.

Connections like these could also lead to new forms of community solidarity. Gerontologist Chris Phillipson has noted the need to recognize what older people bring, as well as receive – their "capacity for civic engagement, support for family and community activities, and distinctive forms of work and education" – through connections that cross generational boundaries. Applewhite came to a similar conclusion: "The sooner we trade the self-sufficiency trap for a more reciprocal, communitarian, age-integrated, mutually interdependent point of view, the closer a truly all-age-friendly society becomes."

FOR THOSE OF US lucky enough, these connections will be among those that sustain us when we are very old. These connections will be with people who know who we are and won't slot us into simplistic ageist categories. But what about those who are not so lucky? What happens, too, when even we lucky ones can't participate in social life in quite the way we once did? It's one thing to build intergenerational relationships and challenge ageist perceptions of frailty and dependence when we are not frail or dependent. But what happens if/when we are? What happens, in other words, when we get to the stage where we need help?

Some things that need to happen are simple structural, "all-age-friendly" fixes. In Applewhite's inimitable terms, there need to be low luggage racks for when we can't hoist suitcases into the high ones. There needs to be more large print, so we can read instructions, and audio assistance for when we can't hear instructions. There needs, in many situations, to be somebody to ask for help – and we need to recognize that, by and large, people like to help. "This culture demands optimism without end, downplays life's challenges, and shames when, inevitably, we fall short," she writes.

It's when we fall short that our self-directed ageism may come to the fore – when we perceive ourselves to be less competent and, therefore, of less value as people, and when we acquiesce to being sidelined or spoken for. In a CBC "Ideas" program on the value of old age that ran in 2021, gerontologist Paul Higgs spoke of our fears about that transition, describing it in terms of a shift from first-person speaking and thinking ("I think that ... ," "I would like ...") to a third-person version ("He is ... ," "She needs ... ," "We will decide ... ," "He'll like that").

At issue is the loss of agency – probably the greatest fear of those of us confronting very old age. One of the people I spoke with said: "Having worked in healthcare, and witnessed both my parents dying ... I would choose to end my life, rather than just dwindle away ... That's where my philosophy lies." Another said: "If things go belly up, I'm out ... If health issues were such that I couldn't live on my own, I would do something about that." A third said: "I could see myself having a cane. I couldn't see myself having a wheelchair." He added: "Staying mobile is the most important thing in my life ... I've said to people, not so jokingly, if I can't walk anymore, I'm going to kill myself. I'm not going to be housebound and dependent on people's care."

In considering the landscape of aging we are now confronting, it's important to note that in June 2016 medical assistance in dying (MAiD) became legal in Canada. In March 2021, some changes to the law came into effect, among them, the removal of the requirement that death be reasonably foreseeable. And pending an expert review, people suffering only from mental illness were temporarily ineligible. Needless to say, medical assistance in dying is an option people might be grateful to draw on.

Bioethicist Erin Gentry Lamb points out that for many people, fear of disability fuels fear of aging. But aging and disability don't always go together. Many people who are not old are housebound and dependent on people's care – and find their lives to be well worth living. What we anticipate about the future may not turn out to be quite as we think. That's not to say there won't be challenges – for us, and for the people we may need to give us care. Respecting personhood when agency seems to be diminishing and help is needed can be a tricky balance. *Negotiating* the help that's needed might not always be easy. But if help is available, and attitudes change, it may not be so hard.

AT THE PERSONAL LEVEL, loss of agency is the issue. Louise was starting to experience this loss when I spoke with her; she was living with recently diagnosed dementia, in a long-term care setting. But the bigger issue is how we think collectively about people like Louise and all the others we now know about, in much worse predicaments, locked away alone in long-term care homes.

In fact, in Canada, older people are more likely to die in long-term care homes than in any other wealthy country. In an interview, André Picard commented on the tendency, in a money-based economy, to see older people as costs and burdens rather than recognizing the lifelong contributions that ought to entitle them to care at the end of their lives. Instead, they are warehoused, as if they no longer matter.

To put it another way, this represents a failure to view older people as citizens with the same human rights as anyone else. In March 2021, a coalition of Ontario advocacy groups was preparing to call on the Ontario Human Rights Commission to undertake an inquiry into systematic discrimination against old people in the province's health care system. Commenting on the move, Anne Levesque, a law professor at the University of Ottawa, described it as exactly the kind of investigation the human rights commission should take on: "This would be the first time that it actually does an inquiry into ageism in our health policies ... I think it's well needed in light of the pandemic ... What are the government's legal obligations toward our aging population, and how can we prevent ageism from influencing government policy and how we treat our seniors?"

When asked in an interview what the first step should be to put things right, Picard responded: "To me, the starting point has to be philosophical. You have to have a philosophy that elders matter, living in the community matters. And after that, if you have a political philosophy, then everything else is pretty well just ... putting into action those philosophies on a practical level."

WHEN IT COMES TO recognizing that elders matter, and that living in the community matters, there's a lot to be learned from Indigenous communities. Elders traditionally are respected and honoured, and their place in the community is not questioned. They are knowledge keepers with memories and stories to tell. But even in these communities, eldercare poses challenges. Dementia is increasing among Indigenous Elders at almost twice the rate of the population at large. That's partly because Indigenous people's health is worse to begin with, with higher rates of diabetes (known to be related to dementia) an important contributor. But the experience of trauma is now also recognized as a factor; tragically, the residential school experience follows Indigenous Elders to the very end of their lives. One Elder who participated in a research study on dementia commented: "Some people choose not to remember."

The broader lesson is the way some Indigenous communities are handling this challenge. For one thing, it isn't always viewed as a tragedy, or a crisis, but rather as part of the circle of life. But where help is sought, it's accepted only on the condition that it's culturally appropriate – not based on treating the individual along the biomedical lines now considered to be the gold standard. Recognition of "Indigenous principles of relationality and interconnectedness" is critical. A remarkable collection of research studies on dementia in

Indigenous communities has recently outlined several approaches (many works in progress, and all devised with Indigenous collaboration) that illustrate how this might be done.

At the broader policy level, change may be coming. Canada may well be influenced by the World Health Organization's new Global Campaign to Combat Ageism, which "aims to change the narrative around age and ageing and help create a world for all ages." And there is now widespread recognition, and the promise of federal funds, to support aging in place – hopefully, as Applewhite puts it, in *all*-age-friendly communities.

Policy shifts such as these, at the broad social level, could be transformative, if they help to bring about change at the interpersonal and personal levels as well. This takes us back to all the public spaces, and the homes, where people of all ages gather and get to know one another. Hopefully, in the course of all this gathering, and the intergenerational connections we establish, ageist stereotypes will diminish, and we will all come to recognize that very old age is part of the cycle of life that, with luck, we'll all experience. We'll recognize that care is something that older people are owed, because they have rights as citizens and because we as a society have a moral duty to care.

Some of us who may be next in line to need that care will need to see ourselves differently, too – not as burdens, diminished by our age, but as important and worthy community members *because* of it.

BABY BOOMERS, ACCORDING to historian Doug Owram, were *born at the right time.* Our luck might be holding – those of us at the front wave might be aging at the right time too.

We lived through exciting times, and tough times, and our experiences haven't all been the same. Some of us have had it much easier than others. But now, in our different ways, we have also lived through a pandemic that has shone a very bright light on the deficiencies in eldercare, which we will soon be needing. It has also highlighted the ageism that has been fundamental to those deficiencies.

So *if* our luck holds – and it is still a pretty big if – change will be coming. Our mission will be to celebrate it and share the benefits, and in the process to create a new model for very old age.

Acknowledgments

When I began to think about writing this book, as a front-wave baby boomer concerned about the (very) old age that was approaching, I knew I would need to talk to a wide range of people with experience of the issues I wanted to explore. It's the way interview projects typically unfold. Finding the relevant experts, and conducting the conversations, is work I find very satisfying. I didn't expect this project to be any different.

But it was – for two main reasons. For the first time, I was working with people with whom I had something important in common. We were all baby boomers, most of us in the older, front wave. While our backgrounds were diverse, we shared a common concern about aging. And that, in turn, created a bond between us that was for me a new experience. I had never before worked with research participants who were as committed, interested, and supportive as this group was. It didn't take long for me to consider them as a team, and to give credit, and thanks, for their significant contributions.

The other difference came about because of the pandemic, which was declared just as I was preparing to end my connection with the participants and get on with writing the book. Instead of pulling back, it seemed important, for many reasons detailed in the text, to follow up with as many of them as were willing to keep in contact. I talked initially to more than a hundred people, across the country, whose backgrounds were as diverse as I could find. They had all agreed to participate in one interview with me, either in person or by phone, Zoom, or Skype, and to allow me to record our conversations. My commitment was to keep the information I gathered confidential. But after that initial interview, most were eager to maintain contact through the strange and troubling pandemic period. Their stories form the heart of this book, and I am so grateful to have been able to use them.

My friend and colleague Liza McCoy also deserves special mention. The support she has given me, on an ongoing basis over many years now, is more than I deserve. She has read every chapter draft, listened to my ideas, and made excellent suggestions. This project, in particular, has greatly benefitted from her support.

Other colleagues and friends have also helped me in many ways. George Campbell, Pat Dunn, Tom Langford, Anne McWhir, Alison Morrow, and Rick Ponting helped me locate potential participants. Val Barr, Fran Burrell, Catherine Kingfisher, and Trish McBride had good ideas, and gave lots of moral support.

I have also been very grateful for the support I have received from UBC Press. It was a pleasure to work with James MacNevin, whose encouragement and excellent advice helped me through some difficult patches. And once the book went into production, I came to appreciate Ann Macklem's input also.

Finally, I would never have made it this far without my family behind me. Thanks to Matt and Caro for their humour, practical help, and sustaining love and support.

Notes

INTRODUCTION

3 **Philip and I met at a Calgary coffee shop**: Philip is not his real name. The names of the people I spoke with, and occasionally other identifying details, have been changed to maintain confidentiality.

6 **stage that one researcher called "encore adulthood"**: Marci Alboher, *The Encore Career Handbook: How to Make a Living and a Difference in the Second Half of Life* (New York: Workman Publishing, 2013); Anne C. Coon and Judith Ann Feuerherm, *Thriving in Retirement: Lessons from Baby Boomer Women* (Santa Barbara, CA: Praeger, 2017); and Phyllis Moen, *Encore Adulthood: Boomers on the Edge of Risk, Renewal, and Purpose* (New York: Oxford University Press, 2016).

6 **Critics of the focus on "successful aging"**: See, for example, Sarah Lamb, ed., *Successful Aging as a Contemporary Obsession: Global Perspectives* (New Brunswick, NJ: Rutgers University Press, 2017); and Jessica E. Pace and Amanda Grenier, "Expanding the Circle of Knowledge: Reconceptualizing the Concept of Successful Aging among Older North American Indigenous Peoples," *Journals of Gerontology: Social Sciences* 72, 2 (2017): 248–58.

6 **"All aging is 'successful'"**: Ashton Applewhite, "Age of Distinction: Don't Believe the Ageist Myths – We Only Get Better in Our Gold Years," *Globe and Mail*, March 3, 2019.

6 **described it as a "black hole"**: Chris Gilleard and Paul Higgs, "Aging without Agency: Theorizing the Fourth Age," *Aging and Mental Health* 14, 2 (2010): 121–28.

8 **roughly equal number of women and men**: My assumption, never contradicted, was that all participants were cisgender adults.

8 **There were also differences:** The group was diverse but not as representative as I would have liked. Not all provinces were represented and – more
critically – there were gaps in the representation of racial and ethnic
backgrounds. In particular, my attempts to find Indigenous Elders willing
to participate were cut short by the pandemic. As future chapters show,
I draw on the work of other researchers to help fill these gaps.

9 **Quebec premier François Legault's March 14 request:** Canadian Press,
"COVID-19: Premier Asked Seniors over 70 to Stay Home," *CTV News*,
March 14, 2021, https://montreal.ctvnews.ca/covid-19-premier-asked
-seniors-over-70-to-stay-home-1.4853281.

9 **By May 25, 2020, 5,324 long-term care residents:** Canadian Institute for
Health Information, *Pandemic Experience in the Long-Term Care Sector:
How Does Canada Compare with Other Countries?* (Ottawa: CIHI,
2020), https://www.cihi.ca/sites/default/files/document/covid-19-rapid
-response-long-term-care-snapshot-en.pdf.

9 **The crisis brought attention:** Paul Moist, "Fast Facts: Canada's Long-Term
Care Workers on the Front Lines of the COVID-19 Pandemic," Canadian
Centre for Policy Alternatives, Commentary, April 6, 2020, https://www.
policyalternatives.ca/publications/commentary/fast-facts-canada
%E2%80%99s-long-term-care-workers-front-lines-covid-19-pandemic.

10 **wide-ranging structural and institutional change in care provision:**
See, for example, Rochelle Baker, "Seniors' Advocates Want National Standards for Care as COVID-19 Surges," *Toronto Star*, November 12, 2021,
https://www.thestar.com/news/canada/2020/11/12/seniors-advocates
-want-national-standards-for-care-as-covid-19-surges.html.

10 **Indigenous communities were also found:** Olivia Stefanovich, "COVID-19
Is Hitting First Nations in Western Canada Especially Hard," *CBC News*,
January 21, 2021, https://www.cbc.ca/news/politics/why-covid19
-spreading-first-nations-western-canada-1.5879821.

11 **contact with care workers to sustain them:** See, for example, Christina
Frangou, "Strict COVID-19 Protocols Are Leaving Seniors Lonely, Depressed and Wondering: Is It Worth It?" *Maclean's*, November 12, 2020,
https://www.macleans.ca/society/health/seniors-covid-19-loneliness
-long-term/.

11 **The availability of social resources:** Charlene H. Chu, Simon Donato-
Woodger, and Christopher J. Dainton, "Competing Crises: COVID-19
Countermeasures and Social Isolation among Older Adults in Long-
Term Care," *Journal of Advanced Nursing* 76, 10 (2020): 2456–59; Briar
Stewart, "Winter Is Already a Trying Time for Some Seniors: COVID-19
Will Make It Worse." *CBC News*, November 27, 2020, https://www.cbc.
ca/news/canada/british-columbia/seniors-isolation-covid-19-winter-1.
5814507.

12 respondents sixty-five years and older planned to support themselves: National Institute of Ageing/Telus Health, "Pandemic Perspectives on Ageing in Canada in Light of COVID-19: Findings from a National Institute on Ageing/Telus Health National Survey," October 2020, https://static1.squarespace.com/static/5c2fa7b03917eed9b5a436d8/t/5f85fe24729f041f154f5668/1602616868871/PandemicPerspectives+oct13.pdf.

12 But neither would we want to be lonely and isolated: See, for example, Stewart, "Winter Is Already a Trying Time."

CHAPTER 1

16 He went on to write a book: Doug Owram, *Born at the Right Time: A History of the Baby-Boom Generation* (Toronto: University of Toronto Press, 1996).

16 Canada saw a 15 percent increase in births: Statistics Canada, "Generations in Canada: Age and Sex, 2011 Census," *Census in Brief*, no. 2, Catalogue no. 98–311–C2011003, https://www12.statcan.gc.ca/census-recensement/2011/as-sa/98-311-x/98-311-x2011003_2-eng.pdf.

17 "the pig in the python": Owram, *Born at the Right Time*, p. x.

17 children in Canada lived with married parents: Nora Bohnert, Anne Milan, and Heather Lathe, "Enduring Diversity: Living Arrangements of Children in Canada over 100 Years of the Census," Demographic Documents, Demography Division, Statistics Canada, April 2014, Catalogue no. 91F0015M–No. 11, https://www150.statcan.gc.ca/n1/en/pub/91f0015m/91f0015m2014011-eng.pdf?st=l3ZrgDTj.

17 "Much of the myth, and hence the power": Owram, *Born at the Right Time*, x.

18 "large events such as depressions and wars": Vern L. Bengston, Glen H. Elder, and Norella M. Putney, "The Life Course Perspective on Ageing: Linked Lives, Timing and History," in *Adult Lives: A Life Course Perspective*, ed. Jeanne Katz, Sheila Peace, and Sue Spurr (Bristol: Policy Press, 2012), 11.

18 "hundreds of thousands grew up": Owram, *Born at the Right Time*, 55.

19 "In earlier generations the predominance": Ibid., 123.

19 "however much the baby boom was a force": Ibid., 159.

20 And though university attendance was much higher: Ibid., 180–81.

20 "This was, after all, 'the' generation": Ibid., 210.

20 The publication in 1962 of Rachel Carson's: Naomi Woodspring, *Baby Boomers: Time and Aging Bodies* (Bristol: Policy Press, 2016), 21.

21 contraception was decriminalized: Canadian Public Health Association, "History of Family Planning in Canada," https://www.cpha.ca/history-family-planning-canada.

21 **homosexuality was also decriminalized**: CBC News, "Timeline: Same-Sex Rights in Canada," *CBC News*, January 12, 2012, https://www.cbc.ca/news/canada/timeline-same-sex-rights-in-canada-1.1147516.

21 **"In some cases, as in the women's movement"**: Owram, *Born at the Right Time*, 306.

22 **the sample had more mobile working lives**: Aneta Bonikowska and Grant Schellenberg, "An Overview of the Working Lives of Older Baby Boomers," Analytical Studies Branch Research Paper Series, October 2013, Social Analysis Division, Statistics Canada, Catalogue no. 11F0019M–No. 352, https://www150.statcan.gc.ca/n1/en/pub/11f0019m/11f0019m2013352-eng.pdf?st=5Tsp3-dE.

22 **Using Canadian census data from 1971 to 1996**: Marie Lavoie, Richard Roy, and Pierre Therrien, "A Growing Trend towards Knowledge Work in Canada," *Research Policy* 32, 5 (2003): 827–44.

22 **More women were working full-time**: Statistics Canada, "The Surge of Women in the Workforce," *Canadian Megatrends*, 2018, Catalogue no. 11–630–X, https://www150.statcan.gc.ca/n1/pub/11-630-x/11-630-x2015009-eng.htm.

22 **Fertility rates began a decline**: Statistics Canada, "Generations in Canada."

23 **under the age of twelve lived in a stepfamily**: Anne Milan, "One Hundred Years of Families," *Canadian Social Trends*, Spring 2000, Statistics Canada, Catalogue no. 11–008–x, https://www150.statcan.gc.ca/n1/en/pub/11-008-x/1999004/article/4909-eng.pdf?st=aDoxX2Us.

23 **Examples included the arrival of**: Statistics Canada, "150 Years of Immigration in Canada," *Canadian Megatrends*, 2016, Catalogue no. 11–630–X, https://www150.statcan.gc.ca/n1/pub/11-630-x/11-630-x2016006-eng.pdf.

24 **"The Indian education system"**: Georgia Carley, "Chanie Wenjack," *Canadian Encyclopedia*, https://www.thecanadianencyclopedia.ca/en/article/charlie-wenjack.

24 **It took until 1996 to close**: "Residential Schools in Canada," *Canadian Encyclopedia*, https://www.thecanadianencyclopedia.ca/en/article/residential-schools.

24 **more than twenty thousand children may have been affected**: Niigaan-wewidam James Sinclair and Sharon Dainard, "Sixties Scoop," *Canadian Encyclopedia*, https://www.thecanadianencyclopedia.ca/en/article/sixties-scoop.

25 **"embedded in relationships with people"**: Bengtson, Elder, and Putney, "The Life Course Perspective," 10–11.

25 **"more tumultuous marriage histories"**: Rachel Margolis, Youjin Choi, Feng Hou, and Michael Haan, "Capturing Trends in Canadian Divorce in an Era without Vital Statistics," *Demographic Research* 41, 52 (2019):

1453–78. See also Western Social Science, "Divorce Data Revealing – and Still Murky," *News and Updates,* February 13, 2020, https://www.ssc.uwo. ca/news/2020/divorce_data_revealing_and_still_murky.html; Rachel Margolis and Youjin Choi, "Divorce and Unpartnered: New Insights on a Growing Population in Canada," research recap, Vanier Institute of the Family, January 19, 2021, https://vanierinstitute.ca/research-recap-divorced -and-unpartnered-new-insights-on-a-growing-population-in-canada/.

25 **high proportion of baby boomers had children:** Rachel Margolis, "The Changing Demography of Grandparenthood," *Journal of Marriage and Families* 78 (2016): 610–22.

25 **some had been grandparents-in-waiting:** Ibid.

25 **boomers have far fewer family connections:** See, for example, Donna S. Lero, "Intergenerational Relations and Societal Change," Vanier Institute of the Family, June 1, 2016, https://vanierinstitute.ca/inter generational-relations-and-societal-change/.

26 **known in the research literature as "elder orphans":** Maria T. Carney, Janice Fujiwara, Brian E. Kemmert Jr., and Barbara Paris, "Elder Orphans Hiding in Plain Sight: A Growing Vulnerable Population," *Current Gerontological and Geriatrics Research,* October 23, 2016, https://doi. org/10.1155/2016/4723250.

26 **households in Canada were single-person:** Statistics Canada, "Families, Households and Marital Status: Key Results from the 2016 Census, *The Daily,* August 2, 2017, https://www150.statcan.gc.ca/n1/daily -quotidien/170802/dq170802a-eng.htm.

26 **housed people over sixty-five:** Jackie Tang, Nora Galbraith, and Johnny Truong, "Living Alone in Canada," *Insights on Canadian Society,* March 6, 2019, Statistics Canada, https://www150.statcan.gc.ca/n1/pub/75 -006-x/2019001/article/00003-eng.htm.

27 **"To an appreciable extent":** Anabel Quan-Haase, Hua Wang, Barry Wellman, and Renwen Zhang, "Weaving Family Connections On and Offline: The Turn to Networked Individualism," in *Connecting Families? Information and Communication Technologies, Generations and the Life Course,* ed. Barbara Barbosa Neves and Claudia Casimiro (Bristol: Policy Press, 2018), 59–80.

27 **fewer connections to younger generations:** Martin Turcotte, "Trends in Social Capital in Canada," *Spotlights on Canadians: Results from the General Social Survey,* May 20, 2015, Statistics Canada, Catalogue no. 89–652–X2015002; and Peter Uhlenberg and Jenny De Jong Gierveld, "Age-Segregation in Later Life: An Examination of Personal Networks," *Ageing and Society* 24 (2004): 5–28.

30 *precarity* **accurately characterized the aging process:** Amanda Grenier, Chris Phillipson, Debbie Laliberte Rudman, Stephanie Hatzifilalithis,

Karen Kobayashi, and Patrik Marier, "Precarity in Late Life: New Forms of Risk and Insecurity," *Journal of Aging Studies* 43 (2017): 9–14. See also Amanda Grenier, Chris Phillipson, and Richard A. Settersten Jr., eds., *Precarity and Ageing: Understanding Insecurity and Risk in Later Life* (Bristol: Policy Press, 2020).

30 **another feature of family (and other) connections:** Toni Antonucci, Kristine J. Ajrouch, and Kira S. Birditt, "The Convoy Model: Explaining Social Relations from a Multidisciplinary Perspective," *Gerontologist* 54, 1 (2017): 82–92; and Heather R. Fuller, Kristine J. Ajrouch, and Toni Antonucci, "The Convoy Model and Later-Life Family Relationships," *Journal of Family Theory and Review* 12 (2020): 126–46.

30 **convoy model builds on work by sociologist Mark Granovetter:** Mark Granovetter, "The Strength of Weak Ties," *American Journal of Sociology* 78, 6 (1973): 1360–80.

CHAPTER 2

32 **Though this multigenerational model of family life:** Nathan Battams, "Sharing a Roof: Multigenerational Homes in Canada (2016 Census Update)," *Transition,* October 2, 2017, Vanier Institute of the Family, https://vanierinstitute.ca/multigenerational-homes-canada/.

33 **Though a high proportion of Canadians:** Rachel Margolis, "The Changing Demography of Grandparenthood," *Journal of Marriage and Families* 78 (2016): 610–22.

34 **"Asking who can be counted on":** Ingrid Arnet Connidis, "Who Counts as Family Later in Life? Following Theoretical Leads," *Journal of Family Theory and Review* 12 (2020): 170.

34 **about two-thirds of Canadians over sixty-five** Sharanjit Uppal and Athanase Barayandema, "Life Satisfaction among Canadian Seniors," *Insights on Canadian Society,* August 2, 2018, Statistics Canada, Catalogue no. 75–006–X, https://www150.statcan.gc.ca/n1/en/pub/75-006-x/2018001/article/54977-eng.pdf?st=JD-V6ZGp.

36 **And their rates of divorce and remarriage:** Rachel Margolis and Youjin Choi, "The Growing and Shifting Divorced Population in Canada," *Canadian Studies in Population* 47 (2020): 43–72. See also Statistics Canada, "Family Matters: Being Separated or Divorced in Canada," Catalogue no. 11–627–M, https://www150.statcan.gc.ca/n1/en/pub/11-627-m/11-627-m2019033-eng.pdf?st=JJfHP-rI; Gretchen Livingston, "Chapter 2: The Demographics of Remarriage," *Four-in-Ten Couples Are Saying 'I Do,' Again,*" Pew Research Center, report, November 14, 2014, https://www.pewsocialtrends.org/2014/11/14/chapter-2-the-demographics-of-remarriage/.

36 **As LAT couples, they are participating**: Ingrid Arnet Connidis, Klas Borell, and Sofie Karlsson, "Ambivalence and Living Apart Together in Later Life: A Critical Research Proposal," *Journal of Marriage and Family* 79, 5 (2017): 1404–18. See also Connidis, "Who Counts as Family Later in Life?"

37 **"a little bit more independent thinking"**: Laura Funk and Karen Kobayashi, "From Motivations to Accounts: An Interpretive Analysis of 'Living Apart Together' Relationships in Mid- to Later-Life Couples," *Journal of Family Issues* 37, 8 (2016): 1113.

37 **"I think a lot of women feel like I do"**: Ibid., 1116.

37 **"The New Reality of Dating over 65"**: Zosia Bielski, "The New Reality of Dating over 65: Men Want to Live Together; Women Don't," *Globe and Mail*, April 27, 2021, https://www.theglobeandmail.com/life/relationships/article-women-older-than-65-dont-want-to-live-with-their-partners/.

38 **In exchange for the dependence on her son**: Prior to 2014, the Family Sponsorship program contained a "ten-year dependency" clause, which required sponsors to provide all the necessities of life to those they sponsored. There were also limits on health care provision and access to basic income programs. See Ilyan Ferrer, "Examining the Disjunctures between Policy and Care in Canada's Parent and Grandparent Super-visa," *International Journal of Migration, Health and Social Care* 11, 4 (2015): 253–67.

40 **"Well, we're friends"**: Ingrid Arnet Connidis and Candace L. Kemp, "Negotiating Actual and Anticipated Parental Support: Multiple Sibling Voices in Three-Generation Families," *Journal of Aging Studies* 22 (2008): 234.

40 **"There were few efforts to share filial responsibility"**: Ibid., 236.

41 **"The reality of an aging population"**: Ibid., 237.

43 **"co-presence across distance"**: Loretta Baldassar, "De-demonizing Distance in Mobile Family Lives: Co-presence, Care Circulation and Poly-media as Vibrant Matter," *Global Networks* 16, 2 (2016): 145–63.

44 **these relationships can be complicated**: See, for example, Lawrence Ganong and Marilyn Coleman, "Studying Stepfamilies: Four Eras of Family Scholarship," *Family Process* 57, 1 (2018): 7–24.

45 **If the two older generations had warm, familial relationships**: Ashton Chapman, Marilyn Coleman, and Lawrence Ganong, "'Like My Grandparent, but Not': A Qualitative Investigation of Skip-Generation Stepgrandchild-Stepgrandparent Relationships," *Journal of Marriage and Family* 78 (2016): 634–43.

46 **And challenges loom ever larger**: Jennifer Baumbusch, Samara Mayer, Alison Phinney, and Sarah Baumbusch, "Aging Together: Caring Relations in Families of Adults with Intellectual Disabilities," *Gerontologist* 57, 2 (2017): 341–47.

47 **Parents' responses are also shaped by family context:** Statistics Canada data suggest that adults living with parents is more common in South Asian and Chinese communities. Both Deepak and Tariq immigrated to Canada from India as young men, and both were still connected to immigrant communities in the cities where they lived. See Vanier Institute of the Family, "In Focus 2019: Adults Living with Parents," fact sheet, February 15, 2019, https://vanierinstitute.ca/in-focus-2019-adults -living-with-parents/.

47 **Researchers now recognize that many family relationships:** See, for example, Ingrid Arnet Connidis, "Exploring Ambivalence in Family Ties: Progress and Prospects," *Journal of Marriage and Family* 77 (2015): 77–95; and Karl Pillemer, Jill Suitor, and Andrés Losada Baltar, "Ambivalence, Families and Care," *International Journal of Care and Caring* 3, 1 (2019): 9–22.

47 **The busy lives of working adults with young children:** See, for example, Gillian Ranson, *The Parents and Children Project: Raising Kids in Canada Today* (Oakville, ON: Rock's Mills Press, 2018).

48 **some thirty-two thousand Canadian children:** Statistics Canada, "Families, Households and Marital Status Highlight Tables, 2016 Census," *The Daily,* August 2, 2017, Catalogue no. 98–402–X2016004, https:// www12.statcan.gc.ca/census-recensement/2016/dp-pd/hlt-fst/fam/index -eng.cfm.

48 **Author Gary Garrison, himself helping to raise step-grandchildren:** Gary Garrison, "The Challenge for All Skipped-Generation Grandparents," *Globe and Mail,* September 28, 2018, https://www.theglobeandmail.com/ opinion/article-the-challenges-of-raising-grandchildren/.

48 **the disproportionate number of Indigenous grandparents:** Jessica Y. Hsieh, Kristen J. Mercer, and Sarah A. Costa, "Parenting a Second Time Around: The Strengths and Challenges of Indigenous Grandparent Caregivers," *GrandFamilies: The Contemporary Journal of Research, Practice and Policy* 4, 1 (2017): 76–114. See also CBC News, "Aboriginal Grandmothers Play Increasing Role in Raising Sask. Children," *CBC News,* November 9, 2015, https://www.cbc.ca/news/canada/saskatoon/aboriginal -grandmothers-play-increasing-role-in-raising-sask-children-1.3311602.

49 **enormous challenges caregiver grandparents face:** Gary Garrison, *Raising Grandkids: Inside Skipped-Generation Families* (Regina: University of Regina Press, 2018).

49 **"I never had that childhood connection with my grandparents":** Grace E. Thompson, Rose E. Cameron, and Esme Fuller-Thompson, "Walking the Red Road: The Role of First Nations Grandparents in Promoting Cultural Well-Being," *International Journal of Aging and Human Development* 76, 1 (2013): 55–78.

49　**about 10 percent of people sixty-five and older:** Rachel Margolis, "The Changing Demography of Grandparenthood," *Journal of Marriage and Family* 78 (2016): 610–22.

49　**much less tolerant of gay parenting:** A 2018 federal government report on social isolation noted that about 50 percent of older LGBTQ people lived without partners, and most did not have children. See Employment and Social Development Canada, *Social Isolation of Seniors: A Focus on LGBTQ Seniors in Canada* (Ottawa: Employment and Social Development Canada, 2018), https://www.canada.ca/content/dam/canada/employment-social-development/corporate/seniors/forum/social-isolation-lgbtq/social-isolation-lgbtq-seniors-EN.pdf.

50　**Ontario's Child and Family Services Act:** Lori E. Ross, Rachel Epstein, Scott Anderson, and Allison Eady, "Policy, Practice and Personal Narratives: Experiences of LGBTQ People with Adoption in Ontario," *Adoption Quarterly* 12 (2009): 272–93.

50　**Family studies scholar Robert Milardo:** Robert Milardo, *The Forgotten Kin: Aunts and Uncles* (Cambridge: Cambridge University Press, 2010).

50　**The term gained some media coverage:** Meagan Campbell, "Canada's Loneliest People: 25 Per Cent of Canadian Seniors Live Alone, but There Lies a Little-Documented Population within That Demographic That Live in Acute Isolation," *Maclean's,* June 22, 2018, https://www.macleans.ca/society/canadas-loneliest-people/; and Angela Mulholland, "Elder Orphans: Childless, Unmarried Baby Boomers Warned to Prepare for Future," *CTV News,* May 15, 2015, https://www.ctvnews.ca/health/elder-orphans-childless-unmarried-baby-boomers-warned-to-prepare-for-future-1.2375440.

50　**heightened risk of loneliness and isolation:** Maria T. Carney, Janice Fujiwara, Brian E. Kemmert Jr., and Barbara Paris, "Elder Orphans Hiding in Plain Sight: A Growing Vulnerable Population," *Current Gerontological and Geriatrics Research,* 2016, https://doi.org/10.1155/2016/4723250/.

50　**pitying, stigmatizing, and ageist:** Bella DePaulo, "Elder Orphans: A Real Problem or a New Way to Scare Singles?" *Psychology Today,* October 4, 2016, https://www.psychologytoday.com/ca/blog/living-single/201610/elder-orphans-real-problem-or-new-way-scare-singles.

CHAPTER 3

55　**81 percent of people aged sixty-five:** Statistics Canada, "Seniors Online," infographic, Catalogue no. 11-627-M, https://www150.statcan.gc.ca/n1/en/pub/11-627-m/11-627-m2019024-eng.pdf?st=dc-FzQgn.

55　**"the great majority of East Yorkers":** Hua Weng, Renwen Zhang, and Barry Wellman, "Are Older Adults Networked Individuals? Insights from

East Yorkers' Network Structure, Relational Autonomy, and Digital Media Use," *Information, Communication and Society* 21, 5 (2018): 681–96.

56 **more socially disconnected than those in other living arrangements:** Xiangnan Chai and Rachel Margolis, "Does Living Alone Mean Spending Time Differently? Time Use and Living Arrangements among Older Canadians," *Canadian Studies in Population* 47 (2020): https://doi.org/ 10.1007/s42650-020-00017-9; E.M Elmer, "Social Isolation and Loneliness among Seniors in Vancouver: Strategies for Reduction and Prevention," report, City of Vancouver Seniors' Advisory Committee, 2018, City of Vancouver and Vancouver Coastal Health, http://www.seniorsloneliness. ca; and Eric Kilinenberg, *Going Solo: The Extraordinary Rise and Surprising Appeal of Living Alone* (New York: Penguin Press, 2012).

57 **phenomenon now called "aging in place":** See, for example, Catherine Donnelly, Paul Nguyen, Simone Parniak, and Vincent DePaul, "Beyond Long-Term Care," *Queen's Gazette*, September 9, 2020, https://www. queensu.ca/gazette/stories/beyond-long-term-care.

58 **data on Canadians' religious affiliation:** See, for example, Pew Research Center, "The Age Gap in Religion around the World," demographic study, June 13, 2018, https://www.pewforum.org/2018/06/13/the-age-gap-in -religion-around-the-world/.

60 **This phenomenon, called *age homophily*:** Peter Uhlenberg and Jenny De Jong Gierveld, "Age-Segregation in Later Life: An Examination of Personal Networks," *Ageing and Society* 24 (2004): 5–28.

60 **meetings happened in age-integrated, shared spaces:** Catherine Elliott O'Dare, Virpi Timonen, and Catherine Conlon, "'Doing' Intergenera-tional Friendship: Challenging the Dominance of Age Homophily in Friendship," *Canadian Journal on Aging* 40, 1 (2021): 73.

61 **older men are less likely to participate:** Mary Anne Nurmi, Corey S. Mackenzie, Kerstin Roger, Kristin Reynolds, and James Urquhart, "Older Men's Perceptions of the Need for and Access to Male-Focused Com-munity Programmes Such as Men's Sheds," *Ageing and Society* 38 (2018): 794–816.

61 **men tend to depend on women:** Ashley E. Ermer and Christine M. Proulx, "Social Support and Well-Being among Older Adult Married Couples: A Dyadic Perspective," *Journal of Social and Personal Relationships* 37, 4 (2020): 1073–91.

62 **a form of masculinity described as "hegemonic":** See, for example, R.W. Connell and James W. Messerschmidt, "Hegemonic Masculinity: Re-thinking the Concept," *Gender and Society* 19, 6 (2005): 829–59.

63 **programming that does exist:** Kristin A. Reynolds, Corey S. Mackenzie, Marie Medved, and Kerstin Roger, "The Experience of Older Male Adults

throughout Their Involvement in a Community Programme for Men," *Ageing and Society* 35 (2015): 531–51.

64 **one of the first Canadian men's sheds:** Ibid.

65 **"Being mainly men is very important":** Ibid., 542.

67 **older immigrant seniors do not always feel comfortable:** Jordana Salma and Bukola Salami, "The Muslim Seniors Study: Needs for Healthy Aging in Muslim Communities in Edmonton, Alberta," University of Alberta, Education and Research Archive, community report, 2018, https://era. library.ualberta.ca/items/ffb80bde-88db-4611-bda6-67ef5108b2bf. See also Jordana Salma and Bukola Salami, "'We Are Like Any Other People, but We Don't Cry Much Because Nobody Listens': The Need to Strengthen Aging Policies and Service Provision for Minorities in Canada," *Gerontologist* 60, 2 (2020): 279–90.

68 **Indigenous seniors who might have experienced trauma:** Employment and Social Development Canada, *Social Isolation of Seniors: A Focus on Indigenous Seniors in Canada* (Ottawa: Employment and Social Development Canada); First Nations Governance Information Centre and Jennifer D. Walker, "Aging and Frailty in First Nations Communities," *Canadian Journal on Aging* 39 (2020): 133–44; and Cyndy Baskin and Caitlin J. Davey, "Grannies, Elders and Friends: Aging Aboriginal Women in Toronto," *Journal of Gerontological Social Work* 58 (2015): 46–65.

68 **concerns about social isolation and a lack of support:** See, for example, Kimberley Wilson and Arne Stinchcombe, "Policy Legacies and Forgotten Histories: Health Impacts on LGBTQ2 Older Adults," policy brief for the House of Commons Standing Committee on Health, May 2, 2019, https:// www.ourcommons.ca/Content/Committee/421/HESA/Brief/BR10449325/ br-external/WilsonKimberley-e.pdf. See also Eric Dicaire, "Gay and Grey in Montreal: How One Group Helps Older LGBTQ+ Crowd Find Community," *CBC News,* January 19, 2021, https://www.cbc.ca/news/ canada/montreal/gay-aging-montreal-pride-1.5875296; and Nick Purdon and Leonardo Palleja, "'We're Going Back into the Closet': LGBTQ Seniors Wary of Being 'Out' in Long-Term Care Facilities," *CBC News,* June 28, 2018, https://www.cbc.ca/news/canada/lgbtq-seniors-long-term-care -homes-discrimination-1.4721384.

68 **"I often think ... is the network around me":** Kimberley Wilson, Katherine Kortes-Miller, and Arne Stinchcombe, "Staying Out of the Closet: LGBT Older Adults' Hopes and Fears in Considering End-of-Life," *Canadian Journal on Aging* 37, 1 (2018): 25.

69 **"We're all just human beings":** Ibid., 26.

69 **older people with disabilities embodied the worst fears:** Emilie Raymond, Julie Castonguay, Mireille Fortier, and Andrée Sévigny, "The Social

Participation of Older People: Get On Board, as They Used to Say!" in *Getting Wise about Getting Old: Debunking Myths about Aging,* ed. Véronique Billette, Patrik Marier, and Anne-Marie Séguin (Vancouver: Purich Books, 2020).

70 **people vary in their needs:** Denise Cloutier-Fisher, Karen Kobayashi, and André Smith, "The Subjective Dimension of Social Isolation: A Qualitative Investigation of Older Adults' Experiences in Small Social Support Networks," *Journal of Aging Studies* 25 (2011): 407–14.

CHAPTER 4

73 **"the steps that can be taken right now":** David A. Sinclair with Matthew D. LaPlante, *Lifespan: Why We Age – and Why We Don't Have To* (New York: Atria Books, 2019).

74 **writer and activist Barbara Ehrenreich:** Barbara Ehrenreich, *Natural Causes: An Epidemic of Wellness, the Certainty of Dying, and Killing Ourselves to Live Longer* (New York: Twelve Books, 2018).

74 **"the emerging scientific case":** Ibid., xv.

74 **"Mostly they understood the task":** Ibid., 2.

74 **"Once I realized I was old enough to die":** Ibid., 3.

75 **"very good or excellent":** See Public Health Agency of Canada, "Aging and Chronic Diseases: A Profile of Canadian Seniors," 2020, https://www. canada.ca/en/public-health/services/publications/diseases-conditions/ aging-chronic-diseases-profile-canadian-seniors-executive-summary. html.

77 **combination of "push" and "pull" factors:** Employment and Social Development Canada, *Report on Housing Needs of Seniors,* June 2019, https://www.canada.ca/en/employment-social-development/corporate/ seniors/forum/report-seniors-housing-needs.html; see also Adam Park and Frederike Ziegler, "A Home for Life? A Critical Perspective on Housing Choice for 'Downsizers' in the UK," *Architecture MPS* 9, 2 (2012): 1–20.

81 **our material convoys:** David J. Ekerdt, *Downsizing: Confronting Our Possessions in Later Life* (New York: Columbia University Press, 2020). See also David J. Ekerdt, "Things and Possessions," in *Ageing in Everyday Life: Materialities and Embodiments,* ed. Stephen Katz (Bristol: Policy Press, 2018).

86 **Sole reliance on government pensions:** See, for example, Richard A. Settersten, "How Life Course Dynamics Matter for Precarity in Later Life," in *Precarity and Ageing: Understanding Insecurity and Risk in Later Life,* ed. Amanda Grenier, Chris Phillipson, and Richard A. Settersten Jr. (Bristol: Policy Press, 2020).

86 Poverty among seniors: Homeless Hub, "About Homelessness," "Seniors," https://www.homelesshub.ca/about-homelessness/population-specific/ seniors.

86 **Canadian social worker Victoria Burns:** Victoria Burns, "Challenging the Myth of Older Homelessness as Chronic Homelessness," in *Getting Wise about Getting Old: Debunking Myths about Aging,* ed. Véronique Billette, Patrik Marier, and Anne-Marie Séguin (Vancouver: Purich Books, 2020).

86 **A combination of financial insecurity:** Karen Kobayashi and Mushira Mohsin Khan, "Precarity, Migration and Ageing," in *Precarity and Ageing: Understanding Insecurity and Risk in Later Life,* ed. Amanda Grenier, Chris Phillipson, and Richard A. Settersten Jr. (Bristol: Policy Press, 2020).

89 **the "most naked" form of precarity:** Gunhild O. Hagestad and Richard A. Settersten Jr., "Aging: It's Interpersonal! Reflections from Two Life Course Migrants," *Gerontologist* 57, 1 (2017): 136–44.

91 **Thanks to a CBC story:** See, for example, CBC News, "Senior Ladies Living Together Group Aims to Help Northern Ontario Women," *CBC News,* March 23, 2019, https://www.cbc.ca/news/canada/sudbury/senior -ladies-living-together-facebook-group-1.5066213; Haydn Watters, "These Seniors Couldn't Afford Living Alone: So They're Becoming Roommates," *CBC News,* May 29, 2019, https://www.cbc.ca/news/canada/toronto/ senior-ladies-living-together-1.5153176; and Joanne Schnurr, "Senior Women Propose Solution to Housing," *CTV News,* October 15, 2019, https://ottawa.ctvnews.ca/senior-women-propose-solution-to-housing -crisis-1.4639243.

CHAPTER 5

97 **major finding of a research study:** Mary L. Sin, Patrick Klaiber, Jin H. Wen, and Anita DeLongis, "Helping Amid the Pandemic: Daily Affective and Social Implications of COVID-19–Related Prosocial Activities," *Gerontologist* 61, 1 (2021): 59–70.

109 **Soaring infection rates in First Nations communities:** See, for example, Christy Somos, "A Year Later, Indigenous Communities Are Fighting Twin Crises: COVID-19 and Inequality," *CTV News,* January 25, 2021, https://www.ctvnews.ca/health/coronavirus/a-year-later-indigenous -communities-are-fighting-twin-crises-covid-19-and-inequality -1.5280843; Kamil Karamali, "How a Toronto Neighbourhood Called a Coronavirus Hotspot Is Pushing Back against COVID-19," *Global News,* December 8, 2020, https://globalnews.ca/news/7510300/thorncliffe-park -coronavirus/; and Erin Anderssen, "Crowded Housing, Tenuous Jobs, and Starting Over in the Midst of a Pandemic Raise Risk of Mental-Health

Issues for Immigrants and Refugees," *Globe and Mail,* June 21, 2020, https://www.theglobeandmail.com/canada/article-crowded-housing -tenuous-jobs-and-starting-over-in-the-midst-of-a/.

110 **large online survey:** Gloria Guttman, Brian de Vries, Robert Beringer, Helena Daudt, and Paneet Gill, *COVID-19 Experiences and Advanced Care Planning among Older Canadians: Influence of Age Group, Gender and Sexual Orientation,* iCAN-ACP Diversity Access Team Report, Simon Fraser University Gerontology Research Centre, January 2021, http:// www.sfu.ca/content/dam/sfu/lgbteol/pdf/FOR%20LGBTEOL%20 Website%20FINAL%20COVID%20ACP%20Report%20Jan%2028 %202021.pdf.

CHAPTER 6

111 **The enterprise was a great success:** Paul Gallant, "How Teaching Urdu to Her Granddaughters Gave Their Grandmother Purpose in a Pandemic," CBC Radio, February 11, 2021, https://www.cbc.ca/radio/white coat/prescription-for-resilience-coping-with-covid-1.5892248/how -teaching-urdu-to-her-granddaughters-gave-this-grandmother -purpose-in-a-pandemic-1.5901869.

115 **Restrictions on in-person contact:** Jackie Tang, Nora Galbraith, and Johnny Truong, "Living Alone in Canada," *Insights on Canadian Society,* March 6, 2019, https://www150.statcan.gc.ca/n1/pub/75-006-x/2019001/ article/00003-eng.htm.

117 **118 people became active daily walkers:** Marcus Gee, "Stepping Up: How One Man's Push to Get His Neighbours Walking Is Starting to Bring a Toronto Community Together," *Globe and Mail,* September 15, 2020, https://www.theglobeandmail.com/canada/article-how-one-mans -push-to-get-his-neighbours-walking-is-starting-to-bring/.

117 **Chapters formed in Toronto:** Shanifa Nasser, "Meet the 9-Year-Old Girl Whose Simple Act of Kindness during COVID-19 Spurred an Army of Volunteers," *CBC News,* April 8, 2021, https://www.cbc.ca/news/canada/ toronto/covid-kindness-good-neighbour-project-hana-fatima-1. 5980113.

117 **Some, like Thelma's group:** See, for example, Kitsilano Cares: COVID-19 Community Support, Facebook public group, https://www.facebook.com/ groups/KitsilanoCares/; and CareMongering: WINNIPEG Community Response to COVID19, Facebook public group, https://www.facebook. com/groups/524262371566511/.

117 **positive media stories might romanticize:** See, for example, Yvonne Su, "Caremongering and the Risk of 'Happy-Washing' during a Pandemic," *Policy Options,* April 14, 2020, https://policyoptions.irpp.org/magazines/

april-2020/caremongering-and-the-risk-of-happy-washing-during
-a-pandemic/.

117 **if they thought help might be needed**: My focus here is on older people living in urban areas since that's where some three-quarters of them live. See Rohan Kembhavi, "Canadian Seniors: A Demographic Profile, research note, Elections Canada, November 2012, https://www.elections.ca/res/rec/part/sen/pdf/sen_e.pdf.

119 **we need weak ties**: Mark Granovetter, "The Strength of Weak Ties," *American Journal of Sociology* 78, 6 (1973): 1360–80.

119 **"Imagine a day that begins"**: Gillian M. Sandstrom and Elizabeth W. Dunn, "Social Interactions and Well-Being: The Surprising Power of Weak Ties," *Personality and Social Psychology Bulletin* 40, 7 (2014): 910.

119 **weak connections have more than passing importance**: Ibid., 919.

120 **"I think often each individual interaction"**: Jonathan Farani, "Why We Need 'Micro-friendships' More Than Ever during the COVID-19 Pandemic," *CTV News*, December 28, 2020, https://www.ctvnews.ca/health/coronavirus/why-we-need-micro-friendships-more-than-ever-during-the-covid-19-pandemic-1.5246535.

120 **social contacts of a diverse array**: Jeffrey A. Hall and Andy J. Merolla, "Connecting Everyday Talk and Time Alone to Global Well-Being," *Human Communication Research* 46 (2020): 86–111. ·

121 **"Small talk is disparaged"**: Moya Sarner, "Lockdown Living: The Social Biome: How to Build Nourishing Friendships – and Banish Loneliness," *Guardian*, March 24, 2021, https://www.theguardian.com/lifeandstyle/2021/mar/24/the-social-biome-how-to-build-nourishing-friendships-and-banish-loneliness?CMP=Share_iOSApp_Other.

121 **The pandemic deprived us**: Farani, "Why We Need 'Micro-friendships.'"

121 **recognition of their value**: Canadian researchers are also picking up on the importance of casual social contacts. See Meg Holden, Atiya Mahmood, Ghazaleh Akbarnejad, Lainey Martin, and Meghan Winters, "Bursting Social Bubbles after COVID-19 Will Make Cities Happier and Healthier Again," *The Conversation*, March 29, 2021, https://theconversation.com/bursting-social-bubbles-after-covid-19-will-make-cities-happier-and-healthier-again-155654.

123 **"COVID-19 Isn't the Only Thing"**: Nathan Stall and Samir Sinha, "COVID-19 Isn't the Only Thing That's Gone Viral. Ageism Has, Too," *Globe and Mail*, March 25, 2020, https://www.theglobeandmail.com/opinion/article-covid-19-isnt-the-only-thing-thats-gone-viral-ageism-has-too/.

124 **concerns were being raised**: James Cairns, *The Myth of the Age of Entitlement: Millennials, Austerity, and Hope* (Toronto: University of Toronto Press, 2017); see also the Generation Squeeze website.

124 **CBC radio program**: CBC On Demand, "Canada Is Unprepared for the Demographic Time-Bomb Hurtling at Us," *The Sunday Magazine with Piya Chattopadhyay,* October 14, 2018, http://www.cbc.ca/listen/shows/sunday-edition/segment/15613808.

124 **"taken their children's future"**: David Willetts, *The Pinch: How the Baby Boomers Took Their Children's Future – and Why They Should Give It Back* (London: Atlantic Books, 2010). See also Max Fawcett, "Will the Boomers Cause a Financial Bust?," *Walrus,* April 9, 2019, https://thewalrus.ca/will-the-boomers-cause-a-financial-bust/.

124 **structural economic changes**: See, for example, John Macnicol, *Neo-liberalising Old Age* (Cambridge: Cambridge University Press, 2015); and Susan Pickard, "Age War as the New Class War? Contemporary Representations of Intergenerational Inequity," *Journal of Social Policy* 48, 2 (2018): 369–86.

124 **Sociologist Jennie Bristow**: Jennie Bristow, *Stop Mugging Grandma: The "Generation Wars" and Why Boomer-Blaming Won't Solve Anything* (New Haven, CT: Yale University Press, 2019). See also Paul Taylor, *The Next America: Boomers, Millennials, and the Looming Generational Showdown* (New York: PublicAffairs, 2014) and Patrik Marier, Yves Carrière, and Jonathan Purenne, "Living on Easy Street? The Myth of the Affluent Senior," in *Getting Wise about Getting Old: Debunking Myths about Aging* ed. Veronique Billette, Patrik Marier, and Anne-Marie Séguin (Vancouver: Purich Books, 2020).

125 **"When this pandemic ends"**: Stall and Sinha, "COVID-19 Isn't the Only Thing That's Gone Viral."

125 **Other media outlets**: See, for example, Ben Waldman, "Pandemic Highlights Widespread Societal Ageism," *Winnipeg Free Press,* October 27, 2020, https://www.winnipegfreepress.com/arts-and-life/life/health/pandemic-highlights-widespread-societal-ageism-572892141.html; and Christina Frangou, "The Year of the Pandemic Has Busted the Myth That Canada Values Its Seniors," *Maclean's,* November 17, 2020, https://www.macleans.ca/society/health/the-year-of-the-pandemic-has-busted-the-myth-that-canada-values-its-seniors/.

125 **group of more than twenty international researchers**: Sarah Fraser et al., "Ageism and COVID-19: What Does Our Society's Response Say about Us?," *Age and Ageing* 49 (2020): 692–95. See also Andrew Wister, "Ageism in the COVID-19 Crisis," *Vancouver Sun,* April 28, 2020, https://vancouversun.com/opinion/andrew-wister-ageism-in-the-covid-19-crisis.

125 **"for purposes of expressing antagonistic"**: Brad A. Meisner, "Are You OK, Boomer? Intensification of Ageism and Intergenerational Tensions on Social Media amid COVID-19," *Leisure Sciences* 43, 1–2 (2021): https://doi.org/10.1080/01490400.2020.1773983.

125 **everyone over a particular chronological age:** See, for example, Eva-Marie Kessler and Catherine E. Bowen, "COVID Ageism as a Public Mental Health Concern," *Lancet* 1, 1 (2020): https://doi.org/10.1016/S2666-7568(20)30002-7.

126 **frequently older adults:** Sally Chivers, "How We Rely on Older Adults, Especially during the Coronavirus Pandemic," *The Conversation,* July 30, 2020, https://theconversation.com/how-we-rely-on-older-adults -especially-during-the-coronavirus-pandemic-143346.

126 **has been labelled "compassionate":** Deanna Vervaecke and Brad A. Meisner, "Caremongering and Assumptions of Need: The Spread of Compassionate Ageism during COVID-19," *Gerontologist* 61, 2 (2020): 159–65.

CHAPTER 7

127 **"we haven't placed a high priority":** CBC Radio, "The Sunday Edition for April 26, 2020," *The Sunday Magazine,* April 24, 2020, https://www.cbc.ca/radio/sunday/the-sunday-edition-for-april-26-2020-1.5536429.

128 **the proportion was about one in four:** Employment and Social Development Canada, *Report on the Housing Needs of Seniors,* June 2019, https://www.canada.ca/en/employment-social-development/corporate/seniors/forum/report-seniors-housing-needs.html; and Statistics Canada, "A Portrait of the Population Aged 85 and Older in 2016 in Canada," May 3, 2017, https://www12.statcan.gc.ca/census-recensement/2016/as-sa/98-200-x/2016004/98-200-x2016004-eng.cfm.

128 **"We did not prepare":** Lindsey Craig, "Ryerson's National Institute on Ageing Pushes for Change in Care of Seniors," *Ryerson Today,* July 14, 2020, https://www.ryerson.ca/news-events/news/2020/07/ryersons -national-institute-on-ageing-pushes-for-change-in-care-of-seniors/.

128 **"the urgent need to improve the lives":** André Picard, *Neglected No More: The Urgent Need to Improve the Lives of Canada's Elders in the Wake of a Pandemic* (Toronto: Random House Canada, 2021).

128 **"Covid-19 exposed a long-standing truth":** Ibid., 48.

129 **The study links the responses:** https://www150.statcan.gc.ca/n1/en/pub/82-003-x/2018005/article/54966-eng.pdf?st=jwMbAPea.

130 **They have had the benefit:** Statistics Canada, "Chronic Conditions among Seniors Aged 65 and Older, Canadian Health Survey on Seniors," Table 13-10-0788-01, January 10, 2021, https://doi.org/10.25318/1310078801 -eng.

130 **they are generally living longer:** Andrew Wister, *Baby Boomer Health Dynamics: How Are We Aging?* (Toronto: University of Toronto Press, 2005).

130　those aged sixty-five to seventy-four: Statistics Canada, "Health Characteristics of Seniors Aged 65 and Over, Canadian Health Survey on Seniors," Table 13-10-0789-01, January 10, 2021, https://doi.org/10.25318/1310078901-eng.

131　"supporting themselves to live safely": National Institute of Ageing/Telus Health, "Pandemic Perspectives on Ageing in Canada in Light of COVID-19: Findings from a National Institute on Ageing/Telus Health National Survey," October 2020, https://static1.squarespace.com/static/5c2fa7b03917eed9b5a436d8/t/5f85fe24729f041f154f5668/1602616868871/PandemicPerspectives+oct13.pdf.

133　"Living in a rural community like Petit Etang": Maxwell Hartt, Samantha Biglieri, Mark W. Rosenberg, and Sarah E. Nelson, eds., *Aging People, Aging Places: Experiences, Opportunities, and Challenges of Growing Older in Canada* (Bristol: Policy Press, 2021), 18–19.

133　nearly three-quarters of people sixty-five: Natalie S. Channer, Samantha Biglieri, and Maxwell Hartt, "Aging in Rural Canada," in Hartt et al., *Aging People*, 180.

133　technology in the form of e-bikes and e-scooters: Jennifer Dean and Edward Donato, "New Micro-mobilities and Aging in the Suburbs," in Hartt et al., *Aging People*, 148–70.

133　When it came to housing: Samantha Biglieri, Maxwell Hartt, and Natalie S. Channer, "Aging in Urban Canada," in Hartt et al., *Aging People*, 34, 38.

134　most older adults in Quebec: Ibid., 40.

134　"There are a few things you need to know": Della Webster and Sylvia Humphries, "Rural Community Vignette," in Hartt et al., *Aging People*, 211.

134　"The ultimate intention of the association": Marrianne Wilkat and Barry Pendergast, with Natalie S. Channer, "Urban Practitioner Vignette," in Hartt et al., *Aging People*, 99.

135　"The facilities that I would like to be in": Lindsay Herman, Ryan Walker, and Mark W. Rosenberg, "An Age-Friendly City? LGBTQ and Frail Older Adults," in Hartt et al., *Aging People*, 123, 132.

135　"These few blocks, these are my village": Catherine E. Tong, Heather A. McKay, Anne Martin-Matthews, Atiya Mahmood, and Joanie Sims-Gould, "'These Few Blocks, They Are My Village': The Physical Activity and Mobility of Foreign-Born Older Adults," *Gerontologist* 60, 4 (2020): 638–50. See also Jordana Salma and Bukola Salami, "The Muslim Seniors Study: Needs for Healthy Aging in Muslim Communities in Edmonton, Alberta," community report, 2018, https://era.library.ualberta.ca/items/ffb80bde-88db-4611-bda6-67ef5108b2bf/view/8b302d89-da05-400c-ba52-066d5053d3a0/MuslimSeniorsStudyCommunityReport_2018.pdf.

135 **"Planners and policy-makers are now playing catch up"**: Mark W. Rosenberg, "Conclusion," in Hartt et al., *Aging People*, 310.

136 **"not necessarily very good at providing"**: Ibid. See also Meghan Joy, Patrik Marier, and Anne-Marie Séguin, "Age-Friendly Cities: A Panacea for Aging in Place?," in *Getting Wise about Getting Old: Debunking Myths about Aging*, ed. Véronique Billette, Patrik Marier, and Anne-Marie Séguin (Vancouver: Purich Books, 2020); Zoltan Varadi, "Civic Infrastructure Ill-Equipped to Serve an Aging Population," *UCalgary News*, n.d., https://ucalgary.ca/news/civic-infrastructure-ill-equipped-serve-aging -population.

136 **"create and be responsible for"**: Rosenberg, "Conclusion," 314.

136 **almost a quarter of seniors lived in unacceptable housing**: Employment and Social Development Canada, *Report on Housing Needs of Seniors*.

137 **A large-screen television monitor assists online interface**: University of Calgary, "Senior Suite of the Future, by UCalgary's Faculty of Environmental Design," YouTube, May 10, 2016, https://www.youtube. com/watch?v=GkoJo9Pg5GQ.

138 **They form part of an expanding universe of digital supports**: Age-Well, "About," https://agewell-nce.ca/.

138 **A report on seniors' housing needs in 2019**: Employment and Social Development Canada, *Report on Housing Needs of Seniors*.

139 **"There's no guarantee adequate home care"**: Picard, *Neglected No More*, 60.

139 **A 2018 policy brief from the Canadian Health Coalition**: Canadian Health Coalition, "Ensuring Quality Care for All Seniors," *Policy Brief*, November 2018, https://www.healthcoalition.ca/wp-content/uploads/ 2018/11/Seniors-care-policy-paper-.pdf.

139 **"The practical implication is that people"**: Picard, *Neglected No More*, 66.

140 **"If you're a senior in this country"**: Ibid., 47.

140 **low-income, racialized, Indigenous, and LGBTQ2S+ seniors**: Canadian Health Coalition, "Ensuring Quality Care for All Seniors."

140 **Many juggled multiple jobs**: See, for example, Paul Moist, "Fast Facts: Canada's Long-Term Care Workers on the Front Lines of the COVID-19 Pandemic," Canadian Centre for Policy Alternatives, Commentary, April 6, 2020, https://www.policyalternatives.ca/publications/commentary/ fast-facts-canada%E2%80%99s-long-term-care-workers-front-lines -covid-19-pandemic; and Naomi Lightman and Courtney Baay, "Will COVID-19 Finally Force Us To Address the Devaluation of Long-Term Care Workers?," *UCalgary News*, n.d., https://ucalgary.ca/news/ will-covid-19-finally-force-us-address-devaluation-long-term-care -workers-0.

140 "Personal care workers are ubiquitous": Picard, *Neglected No More*, 92.

140 "We've got to work really hard to recruit": See Shawn Jeffords, "PSW Pay Gap Hurts Care Services, Advocate Group Says, Calls for More Funding," *CTV News*, March 7, 2021, https://toronto.ctvnews.ca/psw-pay-gap-hurts -home-care-services-advocate-group-says-calls-for-more-funding-1. 5337345.

141 "Most people working in home care": See Julie Ireton, "Home-Care Workers Say Low Wages Are Driving Them Out of the Sector," *CBC News*, March 18, 2021, https://www.cbc.ca/news/canada/ottawa/home-care -workers-poorly-paid-shortage-gender-race-issue-1.5953597.

141 "informally through family or friends": Canadian Health Coalition, "Ensuring Quality Care for All Seniors."

141 caring primarily for their parents or parents-in-law: Statistics in Canada, "Caregivers in Canada, 2018," *The Daily*, January 8, 2020, https://www150. statcan.gc.ca/n1/daily-quotidien/200108/dq200108a-eng.htm.

142 The page includes a video: Employment and Social Development Canada, "Caregiver Readiness: How to Be the Best Caregiver Possible," https:// www.canada.ca/en/employment-social-development/corporate/seniors/ forum/caregiver-readiness-video.html.

142 "One might conclude that while the policy context": Janet Fast, Norah Keating, Jacquie Eales, Chhong Kim, and Yeonjung Lee, "Trajectories of Family Care over the Lifecourse: Evidence from Canada," *Ageing and Society* 41 (2021): 1145–62.

142 "Rather than assume that only those": Ingrid Arnet Connidis, "Who Counts as Family Later in Life? Following Theoretical Leads," *Journal of Family Theory and Review* 12 (2020): 172.

143 personally and financially prepared to become a caregiver: National Institute on Ageing/TELUS Health, "Pandemic Perspectives."

144 Picard's sources put the proportion: Canadian Institute for Health Information, "1 in 9 New Long-Term Care Residents Potentially Could Have Been Cared for at Home," https://www.cihi.ca/en/1-in-9-new-long -term-care-residents-potentially-could-have-been-cared-for-at-home; and Picard, *Neglected No More*.

145 "Municipalities, if they value seniors": Picard, *Neglected No More*, 138.

145 design that makes buildings and communities accessible: See Mississauga, *2015 Facility Accessibility Design Standards*, https://www.mississauga. ca/file/COM/City_Of_Mississauga_Facility_Accessibility_Design_ Standards.pdf; and Calgary, "*Universal Design Handbook: Building Accessible and Inclusive Environments*," https://www.calgary.ca/csps/cns/ publications-guides-and-directories/universal-design-handbook.html.

146 Through collaboration with the Queen's researchers: Catherine Donnelly, Paul Nguyen, Simone Parniak, and Vincent DePaul, "Beyond Long-Term Care: The Benefits of Seniors' Communities That Evolve on Their Own," *The Conversation,* September 8, 2020, https://theconversation.com/beyond-long-term-care-the-benefits-of-seniors-communities-that-evolve-on-their-own-144269.

146 moving in with family members: Picard, *Neglected No More,* 139–42.

146 "whether it's the skill in cleaning": CBC Radio, "The Sunday Edition for April 26, 2020."

147 care worth about \$9 billion in 2019: National Institute on Ageing, *An Evidence Informed National Seniors Strategy for Canada,* 3rd ed. (Toronto: National Institute on Ageing, 2020).

148 "We know we need more jobs in home care": Ai-jen Poo, with Ariane Conrad, *The Age of Dignity: Preparing for the Elder Boom in a Changing America* (New York: New Press, 2015), 119.

149 "The cost of institutional accommodation and care": Don Drummond and Duncan Sinclair, "Enabling Better Aging: The 4 Things Seniors Need, and the 4 Things That Need to Change," *The Conversation,* January 7, 2021, https://theconversation.com/enabling-better-aging-the-4-things-seniors-need-and-the-4-things-that-need-to-change-151191.

149 "After decades of duct tape solutions": Picard, *Neglected No More,* 168.

150 "private or semi-private rooms and bathrooms": Picard, *Neglected No More,* 169.

150 "build a vision of what high quality care": Donna Baines, "Introduction," in *Promising Practices in Long-term Care: Ideas Worth Sharing,* ed. Donna Baines and Pat Armstrong (Ottawa: Canadian Centre for Policy Alternatives, 2019), 12.

150 "The physical integration with the community": Pat Armstrong, "Norway: Small Town. Promising Practices: Community Integration, Great Physical Design, Excellent Food," in Baines and Armstrong, *Promising Practices,* 55.

151 The result was a book: Moira Welsh, *Happily Ever Older: Revolutionary Approaches to Long-Term Care* (Toronto: ECW Press, 2021).

152 "Let's be blunt": Ibid., 209.

CHAPTER 8

154 "I'm tired of the casual ageism in our society": "Don't Assume Seniors Can't Handle Vaccine Booking," reader's letter, *Toronto Star,* March 30, 2021, https://www.thestar.com/opinion/letters_to_the_editors/2021/03/30/dont-assume-seniors-cant-handle-vaccine-booking.html.

154 So those offers of help: Deanna Vervaecke and Brad A. Meisner, "Care-mongering and Assumptions of Need: The Spread of Compassionate Ageism during COVID-19," *Gerontologist* 61, 2 (2021): https://doi.org/10.1093/geront/gnaa131.

155 "the great issue of the next 20 to 30 years": Robert N. Butler, "Dispelling Ageism: The Cross-Cutting Intervention," *Annals of the American Academy of Political and Social Science* 503 (1989): 139.

155 "a deep seated uneasiness": Robert N. Butler "Age-ism: Another Form of Bigotry," *Gerontologist* 9, 4, Part 1 (1969): 243.

156 "Unless we confront these expectations": Ashton Applewhite, *This Chair Rocks: A Manifesto against Ageism* (New York: Celadon Books, 2016), 42.

156 "The sooner growing older is stripped of reflexive dread": Ibid., 60.

156 "We need to stop with the elder apartheid": André Picard, *Neglected No More: The Urgent Need to Improve the Lives of Canada's Elders in the Wake of a Pandemic* (Toronto: Random House Canada, 2021), 178.

156 "Age-friendly communities aren't just wheelchair": Applewhite, *This Chair Rocks,* 180.

157 "odd North American aversion": Elizabeth Renzetti, "My Family Embraced Multigenerational Living: More Canadians Should Do the Same," *Globe and Mail,* December 19, 2020, https://www.theglobeandmail.com/opinion/article-my-family-embraced-multigenerational-living-more-canadians-should-do/.

157 took her to live with them: CBC Radio, "This Couple 'Adopted' Their Elder Friend and Now They Live as a Family," *The Current,* April 29, 2021, https://www.cbc.ca/radio/thecurrent/the-current-for-april-29-2021-1.6006852/this-couple-adopted-their-elder-friend-and-now-they-live-as-a-family-1.6006947.

158 wanting to change the world: See, for example, Karl Pillemer, Linda Wagenet, Debra Goldman, Lori Bushway, and Rhoda Meador, "Environmental Volunteering in Later Life: Benefits and Barriers," *Generations* 33, 4 (2010): 58–63; and Sheri Y. Steinig and Donna M. Butts, "Generations Going Green: Intergenerational Programs Connecting Young and Old to Improve Our Environment," *Generations* 33, 4 (2010): 64–69.

158 A charming video conversation: Anne Karpf, "Don't Let Prejudice against Older People Contaminate the Climate Movement," *Guardian,* January 18, 2020, https://www.theguardian.com/commentisfree/2020/jan/18/ageism-climate-movement-generation-stereotypes.

159 "capacity for civic engagement": Chris Phillipson, *Ageing* (Cambridge: Polity Press, 2013), 167.

159 "The sooner we trade the self-sufficiency trap": Applewhite, *This Chair Rocks,* 180.

159 "This culture demands optimism without end": Ibid., 175–76.

160   **shift from first-person speaking and thinking:** CBC Radio, "Common
      Good: The Value of Old Age," *Ideas,* August 4, 2021, https://www.cbc.ca/
      listen/live-radio/1-23-ideas/clip/15835703-common-good-or-the-value
      -old-age.
160   **fear of disability fuels fear of aging:** Erin Gentry Lamb, "Age and/as
      Disability: A Call for Conversation," Forum, "Age and/as Disability," *Age
      Culture Humanities* 2 (2015): https://ageculturehumanities.org/WP/
      age-andas-disability-a-call-for-conversation-forum-introduction/.
161   **"This would be the first time":** Julie Ireton, "Call for Human Rights
      Inquiry into Health-Care 'Discrimination' of Elderly," *CBC News,* March
      16, 2021, https://www.cbc.ca/news/canada/ottawa/human-rights-request
      -for-inquiry-discrimination-elderly-health-care-ontario-1.5948328. See
      also Elizabeth Payne, "Groups Seek Ontario Human Rights Inquiry into
      Discrimination against Elderly in Health System," *Ottawa Citizen,* March
      16, 2021, https://ottawacitizen.com/news/local-news/groups-seek-ontario
      -human-rights-inquiry-into-discrimination-against-elderly-in-health
      -system.
162   **"To me, the starting point has to be philosophical":** CBC Radio, "André
      Picard on Why We Need a Philisophical Change in Elder Care," *The
      Current,* March 2, 2021, https://www.cbc.ca/listen/live-radio/1-63-the-
      current/clip/15827560-andre-picard-need-philosophical-change
      -elder-care-chefs?onboarding=false.
162   **Dementia is increasing among Indigenous Elders:** Jennifer Walker and
      Kristen Jacklin, "Current and Projected Dementia Prevalence in First
      Nations Populations in Canada," in *Indigenous Peoples and Dementia: New
      Understandings of Memory Loss and Memory Care,* ed. Wendy Hulko,
      Danielle Wilson, and Jean E. Balestrery (Vancouver: UBC Press, 2019).
162   **"Some people choose not to remember":** Barbara Purves and Wendy
      Hulko, "Adapting CIRCA-BC in the Post-Residential-School Era," in ibid.,
      201.
162   **"Indigenous principles of relationality and interconnectedness":** Wendy
      Hulko, Danielle Wilson, and Jean E. Balestrery, "Introduction," in ibid., 7.
162   **remarkable collection of research studies on dementia:** Ibid.
163   **"aims to change the narrative around age and ageing":** World Health
      Organization, "Ageism Is a Global Challenge: UN," news release, March
      18, 2021, https://www.who.int/news/item/18-03-2021-ageism-is-a-global
      -challenge-un.

About the Author

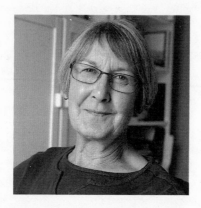

GILLIAN RANSON is a former journalist and professor of sociology. She has written three books on various aspects of family life, inspired by her personal experience as a working mother. Now, as a front-wave boomer and a grandmother, she's exploring aging, and the future she and her peers are likely to find in Canada in the years ahead. She lives in Vancouver.